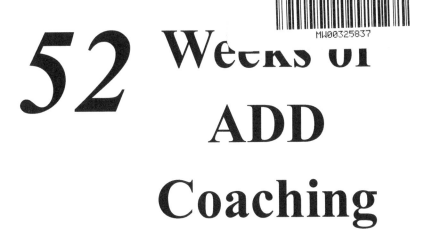

52 Weeks of ADD Coaching

Weekly Empowerment for ADHD/ADD Success & Those who Love Them

By

Dr. Clare Albright

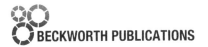

BECKWORTH PUBLICATIONS

Published by Beckworth Publications
3108 E. 10th St.
Trenton, MO 4683
www.BeckworthPublications.com

ISBN-13: 978-0-9847952-3-9

Library of Congress Control Number: 2012932455

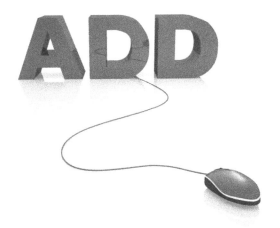

Introduction:

You are about to embark on a journey; a journey that is much like one that you might experience if you were to find yourself in a new and exciting land; someplace you've never seen before.

Shortly after your arrival, you make your way to the active outdoor city market, enjoying the sunshine as it comfortably warms your skin. Suddenly, your attention is captured by the many brilliant colors, the sounds of cheerfulness and joy, and your nostrils are unconsciously flaring, teased by the multifarious aromas wafting through the air around you. Something feels right...something feels very solid about this place.

As you saunter through each market stall, it's almost as if they have been created with you in mind; some more than others. While you find something of value in each of the many shops, some of them call out to you, the sound of your name reverberating contentedly... inviting you to choose from what it has to offer, and to then use your new gift in a manner that is unique to you, and that fits your personality.

You select from these extraordinary places the gifts that appear to be most valuable for what you have in mind, and walk securely away from those that you don't yet indentify with quite as powerfully, knowing full well that should you come back, both the shop, and the particular gift, will still be available and ready for you. This book was written to be a series of shops like the ones described, nestled happily within a metaphorical city market.

In talking and working with countless people - many of them patients - diagnosed with Attention Deficit Disorder (ADD) and Attention Deficit Hyperactivity Disorder (ADHD) over the years, I heard one complaint again and again and again. *"Many of the most potentially useful books on ADD/ADHD, written by supposed experts in these areas, are NOT written in an ADD/ADHD user - friendly way!"*

As I began looking through my own massive library of books on the topic of ADD/ADHD, I found books filled with long chapters... chapters that were 15 - 30 pages in length, each filled with statistics and wordy descriptions using medical terminology.

Personally, I love most of them, and have found many of them to be a godsend; but then again, I've never been diagnosed with ADD/ADHD. Having opted for my doctorate in Clinical Psychology over a quarter of a century ago, I've been conditioned to more easily make sense of what can seem like a mish-mash of gobbled-gook to someone who is simply looking for workable answers and solutions for easing the often frustrating symptoms that accompany ADD/ADHD.

When I examined my personal treasure-trove of ADD/ADHD books through the eyes of someone who is anxiously combing the shelves at the local bookstore seeking, desperately searching, for help, I suddenly found myself looking at stacks of books that were the equivalent of a suitcase packed with one million dollars in cash, but encased in a block of concrete 4 feet thick.

Great ideas are like mental dynamite. When we encounter something that resonates with us deep inside AND can be easily remembered and held firmly in mind (allowing for unfathomable reflection, and, ultimately, application) we are truly standing on transformational ground. This most often occurs in the shadow of simplicity.

This book was written for YOU, the person who has been struggling with ADD/ADHD symptoms. I did not write this book to win the approval of my peers; while I respect them all and appreciate their academic brilliance, trust that their opinion of this book was the farthest thing from my mind. I did not write or structure this book so the critics would have little to pick at. No, YOU are the reason I wrote this book, and it is YOU, and the genius of YOUR brain that this book was designed to connect with. If one or more of my chapters connects with you in a meaningful way, then my venture has been a successful one, and so has yours.

It is an honor, an absolute honor, to be able to share these ideas with you. I wish you well.

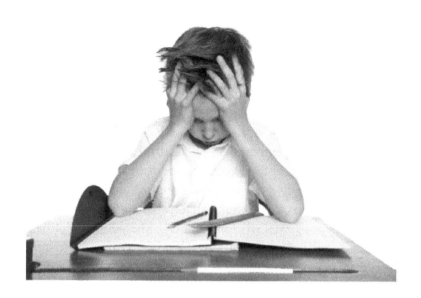

Chapter One:
Grades Were About the Class, Not You

"Hard work is more important than genetic high intellect in achieving success."

- Thomas J. Stanley.

Most of the adults I've met who were diagnosed with ADD/ADHD as children have a less than stellar track record when it comes to academic performance. However, it's not the grades that were stamped on their report cards that are problematic today. Far more destructive than any grade they received are the beliefs they have about what those grades meant about them, and the identity they had established based on those beliefs.

Let me be clear about something; anyone who has worked hard for a high grade point average should be proud of their accomplishments. With that being said, things like a high SAT score, or being a straight "A" student are very much overrated when it comes to business, professional or financial success. In fact, the most successful people in these areas are usually *not* the ones with the highest SAT scores or GPA. Shocked? Most people are.

In his book "The Millionaire Mind," Thomas J. Stanley shares what his years of research revealed about millionaires who received low grades while in school. While those around them with low grades allowed the grade to determine "who" they were, the future millionaires refused to buy into the dogma put forth by the educational system that, unless you could get good grades consistently, you stood little chance at success in the world. Instead, they forged their own path, and chose to view the low scores as what they were - low scores - and nothing more.

If you brought home nothing but "A's" on your grade cards, or were a 4.0 student in college; great. If not, remember this: SWSWSW. That stands for *"Some will, some won't, so what?"* Einstein and Edison were both poor students. Was their academic performance an accurate predictor of what they would contribute to the world? Hardly.

Here's what I know about you. When you are interested and passionate about what you are studying or learning, you'll do well - extremely well. When you are not, it will take a great deal of focus and determination to do well. Not that you can't, or won't do well, it will just take more effort. Are you beginning to see the answer to this challenge? One critical element of all successful ADD/ADHD folks is that they stopped trying to fit a square peg in a round hole. They discovered the area for which they had the "fire in the gut" and then focused their attention (quite effortlessly) in that area.

Michael Neill says, *"you want what you want, whether you think you can have it or not."* What do you want? What makes you tick? Just as you would never try to drive forward by looking only into the rear-view mirror, neither should you make your way through life by looking to your past accomplishments or academic performance. What you had done, or scored, says nothing about now.

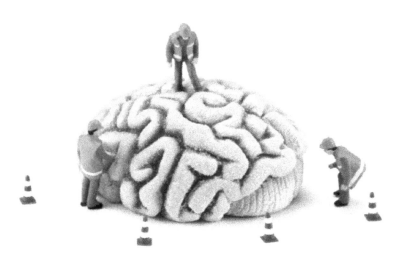

Chapter Two:
Instantly Eliminate Limiting Beliefs
About ADD/ADHD

"You can have anything you want if you will give up the belief that you can't have it."

- Dr. Robert Anthony.

Just what is a belief? A belief is nothing more than a feeling of certainty about a particular idea or concept. The more intense the feeling of certainty, the stronger the belief. The stronger the belief, the more influence it exerts in one's life and the decisions we make.

While I have no idea what the beliefs you hold about ADD/ADHD are, this much I do know... you have beliefs about what ADD/ADHD is and what it means to you. When we have a limiting belief, the belief itself is enough to prevent us from making progress.

If I have the belief *"ADD/ADHD is genetic, so there's nothing I can do about it,"* then I won't attempt to do anything about it, or improve the situation in any meaningful way. Beliefs can become self-fulfilling prophecies; if I believe it's genetic, and there's nothing I can do about it, I don't try to do anything about it. Because I don't try to do anything about it, nothing changes or improves. Because nothing changes or improves, my belief gets even stronger. *"It's true, there's nothing you can do about it,"* I argue. *"Nothing has changed in 15 years!"* Do you see how this insidious cycle works to keep you stuck, feeling helpless?

The way out of this loop is straightforward and simple. You won't find much "peer-reviewed" research on the method I'm going to show you, but I can tell you that the proof you are looking for will be found in the proverbial "pudding"; use the method I show you, and you'll find how easily it works to destabilize limiting beliefs.

This method was shared with me by "America's Body Language Guy", and author of *The Productivity Epiphany,* Vincent Harris. He has been coaching and consulting high-level clients for 11 years now, and rates this method as one of his most reliable tools for pulling the plug on a client's shoddy beliefs.

Years from now, when the effectiveness of this "new" method for working with beliefs is finally approved, you will happily be able to say *"Oh, THAT one; I was using it years ago!"*

What this method does is cause you to feel less certainty - even uncertainty - about something you had previously felt with a great deal of conviction. It's really as simple as that. Think about it; at one time, you believed in the Easter Bunny - you felt certain about the idea he existed.

One day, however, you were introduced to contradictory information - perhaps you witnessed your parents setting out the Easter eggs - and suddenly, the feeling you had about the existence of the Easter Bunny destabilized, and you were left with a very uncertain feeling - one full of doubt - when you heard someone talk about the hippity hoppity rabbit.

Now, years later, you sometimes feel silly, wondering how you could have ever believed in an over-sized rabbit that hops around the globe leaving treats for children. But the most significant change is how it impacted your behavior. Because you no longer felt certain, you stopped going to bed with excitement, and lunging out of bed to check for goodies. You didn't have to do "affirmations" to get yourself to stop a tradition many years old... you simply changed a belief and voila!... instant behavioral change. Who'd a thunk?

Here are the simple steps for pulling the rug out from underneath any belief that's no longer (or perhaps never was) serving you well:

1. **Identify the limiting belief**: The easiest way to do this is to simply start listening to the comments you make, both to others, and internally to yourself. Whenever you hear yourself say something that sounds like a possible limiting belief, ask *"How does using this belief as something to guide me through life impact my behaviors?"*
2. **Destabilize the Belief:** The certainty of many ideas is held in place by the images, sounds, smells, tastes and feelings that congregate inside your mind to complete the picture.

So, what you will be doing is "scrambling" the sensory data related to the belief you have identified, and would like to obliterate. You will do this in three primary sensory channels. Just as we have three primary colors to mix and create other lovely hues, the senses of sight, sound and feeling are so central to the formation of most ideas, that they and they alone, can tame the wildest of them.

Once you have identified the belief, and are prepared to destabilize it, you're ready to use a simple 1.2.3 approach to get down to business.

It goes like this: While you are holding the thought of your belief in mind (don't worry about 'doing it right'... as long as you are thinking about the belief - however it is that YOU think of it, this will work like a charm). You are going to simultaneously move your eyes, hum a silly song, and tap on your forehead.

Move your eyes in erratic and irregular patterns; up and down, side to side, diagonal, figure 8's, circles, zigzags... just keep changing every 3 - 5 seconds. For the song, pick something silly; I like the circus music personally, but others like "Scooby-Doo", "The Adam's Family" theme song, etc. The important thing is that you pick something that, when you think about it, or sing/hum it, you just can't be too serious. Finally, at a rate of 2 - 3 taps per second, you'll be tapping on your forehead, just between your eyebrows.

You'll want to do all three (eyes, song and tapping) simultaneously for about 30 seconds at a time. Just rate the degree of certainty you feel about the belief before you begin (scale of 1 - 10) and then begin, doing your best to hold the belief in mind for the entire 30 seconds. When you've stopped, rate the certainty again, and repeat this process until your level of certainty is only 1 - 3.

You can sing the song out-loud, inside your head, or you can hum; it makes no difference.

Here's what I know about beliefs: as you begin eliminating the ones that have been causing you to think, feel and behave in a prejudicial manner, your life will change, and any other method you use will work more easily and effortlessly.

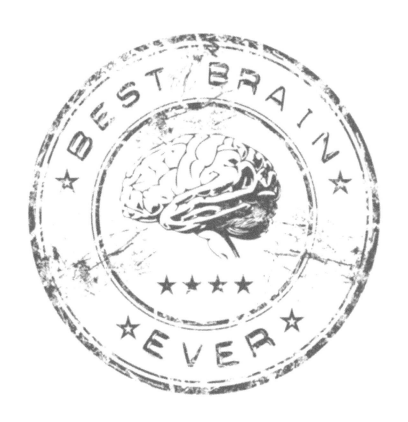

Chapter Three:
Going from "Attention" to "Attending"

"Perfection has to do with the end product, but excellence has to do with the process."

- Jerry Moran.

I'd like you to consider something; I'd like to send you a small box of attention. Attention is not a hazardous material, so, even if you happen to live overseas, it's nothing a simple customs form won't take care of. Do you have a place in mind where you'll put your gift when it arrives?

Attention might look good on a shelf, or perhaps a night stand next to the bed?

Are you somewhat confused? I sure hope so. *"Attention" isn't a noun - a person, place, or…that's right…it is not a "THING"*!

Does it seem like I'm splitting hairs? I am. In a moment, you'll see why. It has to do with a process called "nominalization".

By definition, a nominalization is when we take a verb - a process - and alter its structure, making it sound very much like a noun. When this happens, strange things happen to us neurologically.

Have you ever had a bad relationship? Wheeww… fixing a "thing" like a relationship can seem like an insurmountable task. Can you set a relationship on an end table? No? Ahhh, then it may very well be a nominalization. Lets track relationship back to the verb it was born of, and lo and behold, we find "relating".

If you and I are relating poorly at any given moment and suddenly change the manner in how we are relating, the experience we are having changes just about as suddenly. However, if we think about our turmoil as a "bad" relationship - a "thing" - we may find that we immediately think and feel as though we have a situation that will take weeks of therapy or counseling to "fix".

Let's examine "Attention". I think you'll agree, you cannot place attention in a container, or hold it in your hand and pass it around the room for others to look at. When we track it back to "verb land" we find "attending" - a process in a constant state of flux.

You and I are always attending to something. It's not as if our brain shuts off when we are no longer attending to the project that is on our desk; even if it appears to others that we are in a zombie-like state, our eyes fixed straight ahead and our arms near cataleptic, it's always a matter of what are we attending to in any given moment.

In this case, it's likely that we are attending more to the sights, sounds and images in our mind (day dreaming), than we are to those in our external environment. There is no "Attention Deficit", I would argue, there is simply the case of attending to something other than what would be more beneficial for us to attend to at any given moment.

Some parents will tell me, *"my son has severe Attention Deficit Disorder; he totally ignores his homework and gets lost in that damn video game!"* I'm thinking, *"So, this kid with a supposed Attention Deficit can attend to, and focus on, a video game so successfully, that nothing else has the ability to distract him? That seems like a wonderful gift to me; let's see what other areas of his life we can get him to attend to like that!"*

My point is simple. When we mistakenly come to view an ongoing process as a fixed and static "thing", we will no doubt fail to see many of the otherwise obvious possibilities that exist. Once I understand that "attending" is something I do, I automatically begin to feel a much greater sense of control. However, once I have been conditioned to think of myself as someone who is lacking something (attention), it's easy to assume that I am somehow "broken" and must therefore be "fixed".

Remember, words are labels to describe an experience, but they will always fall short of conveying the experience they describe accurately. However, once we have started using a given way of talking about, and thinking of an experience, the words we use actually begin to shape how we process that experience, thus "attention" feels like something that will be hard to work with. Conversely, "attending" radiates movement, hope and the ability to do something that will make a difference.

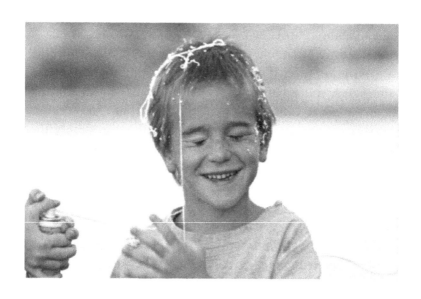

Chapter Four:
Calm Down? Why?

"There are only two ways to live your life. One is as though nothing is a miracle. **The other is as though everything is a miracle.**"

- Albert Einstein.

Many people have tired of hearing others say, *"You need to calm down; you are always too hyper and unable to focus on anything!"* The implication is that hyperactivity is counterproductive and is therefore "bad". This usually has more to do with how the non ADD/ADHD person making this statement feels *about* someone's hyperactivity, and has very little to do with the "truth" of the matter.

In 1986 a study looked at the most creative students and found something that may, or may not, come as a surprise to you. Those scoring the highest on creativity were also found to be a great deal more hyperactive. They talked faster, fidgeted more, and had an abundance of energy.

It's really easy to get caught up in what we can't do because of our hyperactive nature. I have a question for you, though; what are the things you *can* do, and do well, *because* of your hyperactive nature? Once you have identified the things you have done because of it, all of a sudden, you find an interesting shift occurring; now, instead of seeing it as a curse, you begin to feel a little anxious about the thought of "losing" this precious gift.

Do you realize - truly realize - how many people grumble and complain each day about not having enough energy? Men and women around the world struggle just to get the most fundamental tasks done each day; paying bills, washing dishes, ironing clothes, etc. The thought of "brain storming" about colorful and vibrant new ideas and action plans is just too much. Sadly, many people hope to have enough energy to make it through one more arduous day and safely into bed where they will strive to re-charge for yet another taxing round of life. Sound like fun?

Begin to think of hyperactivity as an abundant - almost endless supply - of energy. Would you rather have a road map of where you were going, but no gas in the tank, or a full tank of gas and some idea of where you were going? With a full tank of gas, you can do the most important part; you can get started! With the energy to begin, you can ask others along the way for directions and, as long as you have enough gas, you'll get there. Without gas in the tank, though, I don't care how clear your directions are. You have a gift; the key is to channel it!

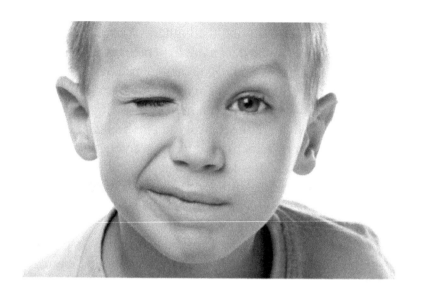

Chapter Five:
You Don't Have to Finish
Everything You Start!

"To me success means effectiveness in the world, that I am able to carry my ideas and values into the world - that I am able to change it in positive ways."

- Maxine Hong Kingston.

Since you are reading this, either you, or someone you love has a highly creative mind; almost everyone diagnosed with ADD/ADHD is very creative and generates lots and lots of new ideas. Since there are only so many hours in the day though, it stands to reason that there will be more ideas born, and more projects started than you will actually have time to see through to completion.

Is this a problem? I suppose it *can* be, but more times than not, the real problem is the stress people experience when they realize, *"I've got so many projects going on and I'll never get them all done."* There is, of course, with this kind of thinking, an underlying belief that says we *have* to finish everything we start.

What I'm proposing is going to run counter to most everything you've ever been told:

Forget about finishing everything you start; it is a goal that will only cause you undue stress and keep you from completing the things that really are important.

When others suggest that you should "always finish what you start" they are not taking into consideration the way your brain works. You generate an abundance of wonderfully creative and unique ideas. If you are honest with yourself, some of them are nothing short of brilliant and, many of them, are pretty wacky and useless once you've had a chance to think about them.

Thomas Edison is known for the light bulb. We've all heard the story about his thousands of "failures" and the tenacity he demonstrated when he was working to find the right filament for the bulb. From this, we are led to believe that Edison, once he started something, never wavered, and saw everything he started through to the end.

What we don't hear about, though, are all of the experiments that Edison abandoned. See, Edison knew the power of stopping from time to time to ask the question, *"Is this still as important to me as it was when I started?"* If it was, then he would knuckle down and proceed... even if he had fallen behind schedule. If his answer was "no" however, he would immediately drop it from the list. Why do something for the sake of doing it, if it's no longer important?

Know this; as quickly as your mind works, there will be many things you start, that simply don't hold the same importance to you a short time after you have started. Stop beating yourself up about "finishing everything", and focus on finishing the important things and dropping everything else. You'll be amazed at what happens.

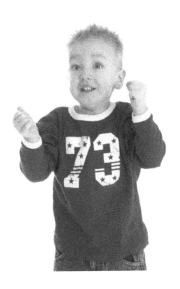

Chapter Six:
The "Holy Grail" Trap

"General Systems Theory, a related modern concept [to holism], says that each variable in any system interacts with the other variables so thoroughly that cause and effect cannot be separated. A simple variable can be both cause and effect. Reality will not be still. And it cannot be taken apart! You cannot understand a cell, a rat, a brain structure, a family, a culture if you isolate it from its context. Relationship is everything."

- Marylin Ferguson.

Time and time again, whether it be someone who is dealing with Attention Deficit Disorder (ADD), Attention Hyperactivity Deficit Disorder (ADHD), Chronic Pain, Depression, or an almost unlimited number of other unsavory situations, we see people who move from one thing to another, in search of the "one" thing that will magically and quickly bring the relief they have been seeking.

Why do so many go searching for what I call the "Holy Grail"? It may very well spring forth from the underlying belief that many of these conditions have one, and only one, cause. Although this might turn out to be true in some cases, in the vast majority, this is not necessarily so.

What we do know at the current time, however, is that there is not a universally agreed upon cause for ADD/ADHD. Single cause for Strep throat? Yes; this can easily be determined with a swab of the affected area and, once identified, the appropriate antibiotic can be prescribed to eliminate this single known cause of the condition we've come to refer to as "Strep Throat". To date, though, there is no such test for ADD/ADHD.

Oh, you can be sure that many in a wide range of specialty areas will claim to know the cause of ADD/ADHD. It's not uncommon for an EEG Biofeedback Specialist, Chiropractor, Herbalist, Physiotherapist, Psychologist, Nutritionist, etc., to profess to know the "real" cause of these conditions and, as you might have guessed, it just so happens that their particular area of specialty holds the only "true" cure or relief.

Now, let me be clear about something; I am a licensed and practicing psychologist and a certified EEG Biofeedback clinician. I have seen people improve tremendously after using EEG Biofeedback or Neurofeedback.

I have also seen people make a great deal of progress with their ADD/ADHD by taking certain nutritional supplements, cutting things from their diet, getting Chiropractic care, or after a number of sessions with a skilled hypnotherapist… I have seen them all work for *some* people, but

I have not seen, nor does the research suggest, that *any* of them help *all* people with ADD/ADHD.

The problem, as I see it, is that once someone has used any particular method in an attempt to deal effectively with their aggravating symptoms, and do not meet with the *"Oh my God!"* earth-shaking results they had hoped for, they quickly scrap the whole thing, and then rapidly move to the next potential "miracle".

There is a particular pot roast recipe that I'm fond of. For spices, it includes ginger, garlic, poppy seeds, salt, rosemary, turmeric, cumin, bay leaves, red pepper flakes and cloves.

If I were to cook my roast with only salt, for example, I might conclude that "salt" does not "work" and decide to discard it as a possible flavoring for my dinner. In fact, any of the spices I use in my recipe, by themselves, would probably leave a great deal to be desired. Together, however, they coalesce to create a flavor that cannot be produced by any one spice alone, but that can only be enjoyed after the collective flavors have merged.

I am proposing that you may find my "pot roast" metaphor a useful way to think about the many wonderful options that exist to move you from where you are now to where you want to be - or at least really close to it.

EEG Biofeedback may, or may not, give you the complete relief you had hoped for, and a specific nutritional supplement may not do the trick, but the chances are very good indeed, that you'll find several things that will help in some way, to varying degrees. When you employ them all - simultaneously - the symptoms that had once plagued you may slowly - or quickly - become a distant memory.

I urge you to set aside - at least temporarily - the belief that ADD and/or ADHD have only one cause, and only one "true" method of treatment and, instead, begin to get curious, asking *"what methods can I use, and in what combination can I use them, that will allow me to move beyond the bothersome symptoms of ADD/ADHD and into a more focused and productive realm of life?"*

I believe this mind set, or manner of thinking about your current situation, will allow you to find your own "recipe"; a collection of two or more things that will have you one day looking back and noticing just how far you've come, and how much happier you are.

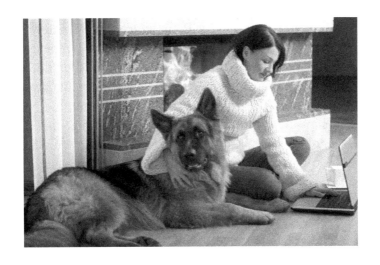

Chapter Seven:
Finding Your Home

"Do what you love. Know your own bone; gnaw at it,
bury it, unearth it, and gnaw it still."

- Henry David Thoreau.

Roger Daltrey, former lead man of the world famous rock band "The Who", is on tour as a solo artist. He's 66 years old, an age when many are well into their first year of retirement, having escaped a job or career they despised for 20 - 45 years or more. He still sings with vigor and passion, touring around the world. It's certainly not for the money.

Same thing with Sir Paul McCartney, with an estimated net worth of 500 million dollars, Sir Paul could have easily settled into a life of a comfortable recliner and day after day of television long ago.

Why do Roger and Sir Paul, who are legitimately senior citizens now, continue with the travel, the rehearsals and the nightly performances? They do what they do, because they love what they are doing, and don't look at what they do as work. It's really just as simple as that.

Think of some hobby you have; the thing that you think about all day, and can't wait to do when you get off work. Do you ever think about how many more years you have to go until you get to retire from golf, or whatever your passion may be? Of course not, that would be ludicrous.

That's exactly how someone like Daltrey or McCartney think about performing; why would they think about when they can stop doing what they love doing?

Few things make life for someone diagnosed with ADD/ADHD more frustrating than getting up every day and trudging off to a job that they don't enjoy. Many spend every moment at work trying to somehow compensate for the boredom by doodling, daydreaming, or some other method of self-stimulation.

They constantly check their watch, looking to see how many more hours, minutes or seconds until they will be "set free" and will step out of the confining environment with too many restrictions and rules to be able to express their creativity and unique way of doing things.

No matter how unique or specific your hobby or area of passionate interest may be, we now live in an era of connectivity that allows you to earn a living - often a very good living - doing exactly what you used to do only as a hobby, and for no pay. With the internet and social networking, it is now possible to tap into the other people in the world who share a deep interest in the same area.

Begin now, to look at the obvious. What do you love to do? Forget about asking whether it's possible to transform this into a business or income at this point, just identify it first. Then, once you know what it is, start to ask the question, *"How many ways can I find to earn an income with this?"* Once you ask that question, and begin an honest search for the answers, you'll find them.

You've got one shot at this life and you've also been blessed with a gift (if you harness it) to utilize during your time on planet Earth. The question is, are you going to milk it for all it's worth and enjoy it, or will you choose to focus on how you are different and "deficient"?

I know it sounds way too simple, but that's because it is; find what you like, and do everything you can to earn a living that way.

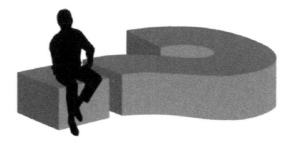

Chapter Eight:
Delegate and Outsource to Make Better Use of Your Time and Get More Done

"Every person I work with knows something better than me. My job is to listen long enough to find it and use it."

- Jack Nichols.

Success is not difficult to achieve and no achiever is without some sort of shortcoming. You think "*I have ADD/ADHD and I'll never be able to do as much as so and so*", or "*It is impossible, I just can't do this job, because I have ADD, I shouldn't take it on*". You see the defeatist attitude you put before yourself, even before you can actually start the work you have to do.

I bet you have read several books which talk about how the universe comes together to give you what your heart desires if you wish for it and work hard enough. Wishing well before the start of your project might not get your work done for you; but it will surely place you in a receptive frame of mind. Talking of mind, this mind of ours has a strange way of working. Have you noticed how we often receive what we perceive? If we perceive failure, more often than not, that is what we get. Same goes for success. So, start it off on a good note.

Now, I don't mean that you should keep taking on work. Recognizing and accepting your shortcomings and being realistic about what you can possibly do is the key to achieving completion and satisfaction. But you might wonder, *"Job completion, satisfaction and all that is fine, but I want to be able to do more with my time"*. It is understandable that the productivity of an ADD/ADHD individual will not be as good as that of a non-ADD/ADHD one. Low concentration and a distracted mental state tend to bring down productivity. The key here is to find a way to work around these ADD-associated characteristics.

Let's look at Bill Gates, who needs no introduction and has a net worth of $53 billion as of 2010. Microsoft is an impossibly huge company today and as is well known across the globe; Gates is a school dropout. How do you think Microsoft came about? Did Gates make each and every program that came out of Microsoft's doors or "windows"? Absolutely not. What he did was delegate and outsource.

There are people out there who can do your work for you, so assign them part of your work. No CEO does all the work by himself, in fact he might only delegate. Master that art. So what if you can't be the worker bee and find nectar, you can surely be the queen bee, capable of having indisputable power over all the worker bees. Proper delegation will ensure you get more done in a day than you would have in a week if you did it alone.

You know that tomorrow never comes, but your procrastination refuses to leave you. Imagine you've been told to write and direct a play, one which is scheduled within the next month. Now, although you love directing and it brings out the creative side in you, writing the play is of no interest to you. Outsource your work. There are people out there who will do it for you, the way you want it. Pay them commensurate to the work they do. It will be an investment which will pay you back manifold.

Follow the POD rule for increased productivity: Plan, Outsource and Delegate. There are certain requirements you need to fulfill before you become a master delegate or outsourcer. First and foremost, learn to trust. It is only when you are able to trust the person before you to do the job you want, that you will be able to assign him or her the work. But trusting blindly has its pitfalls. So, learn to judge. Learn to separate the good from the bad, the trustworthy from the deceitful, from the little information you might have to get going. Learn to encourage. You are human; they are human too. You procrastinate and so do they. But encouragement goes a long way in ensuring timely completion of your job.

The POD rule will ensure that the work that would have previously overwhelmed you fails to do so anymore and you end up achieving a lot more each day than you would have otherwise. It will ensure that your ADD does not restrict your productivity and you go to bed feeling successful each day.

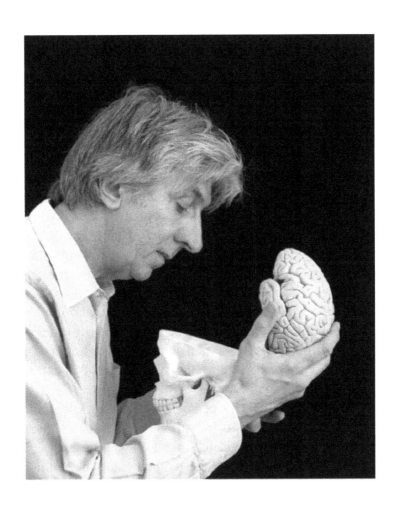

Chapter Nine:
Expect a letdown after success

"Nothing recedes like success."

- Walter Winchell.

In the several years of my experience with treating ADD/ADHD persons, there is one trend I've noticed that continues to surprise me. Many individuals complain of feelings of depression following success of any sort. Paradoxical as it sounds, I have noticed this swift dip after a rise in umpteen cases and cannot disregard it.

Mood swings, lack of concentration, inability to focus, and procrastination characterize ADD/ADHD. It is therefore no wonder that each success that comes your way was one earned by hard work of the highest degree. Success does not come easy, especially for an ADD/ADHD individual.

Think Thomas Alva Edison. In his own words: *"Results? Why, man, I have gotten lots of results! If I find 10,000 ways something won't work, I haven't failed. I am not discouraged, because every wrong attempt discarded is often a step forward."* You see the number of times he must have gone wrong? When something goes right after you've faced several failures, the high that you will experience is understandable.

Most ADD/ADHD persons who do not often find themselves in successful situations, experience a steep pinnacle of emotions and feelings following a successful venture. Equally drastic is the way their emotions plummet deep enough to cause depression-like symptoms.

Sometimes, a successful venture is not the only thing that can cause this hillock; this mountain of feelings. Win or lose, ADD/ADHD patients go for the thrill. The excitement of the chase as you work towards your goal can get a little addictive. When the venture ends and the excitement and high are gone, depression takes over.

What can you do when you know about the unavoidable future occurrence of a distasteful event? Prepare yourself. Be ready to face it when it comes; don't let it take you unawares.

Regions near the Tundra are graced with snowfalls for the major part of the year. One moment they will be in the midst of summer and the next they are catapulted into winter. The animals that can survive the biting cold, trudge on, but what about the smaller ones? They are prepared, always, for a turn of events; from bright, warm and cheerful to dark, cold and stormy. They hibernate through the winter months and emerge next summer.

I am not asking you to go into hibernation following each success. They are animals, acting as nature ordained them to. We, on the other hand, are humans with a mind of our own. Move on to the next big venture. If you stop long enough to begin missing the feeling of having something big to do, you'll end up feeling depressed.

If Thomas Edison had stopped to get depressed after each of those 10,000 mistakes he made, he would not have had the 1,090 odd patents to his credit. What the heck, he wouldn't even have had enough time to make 1,000 mistakes or invent 10 things, if he dedicated time after each success and failure to thinking depressive thoughts.

Try this the next time you complete something successfully and are feeling happy and successful. Sit down in a quiet place and have a heart-to-heart with yourself. Tell your mind what's to come; the depression-like feelings and the sense of loss.

This may sound stupid to you, but it isn't. Have you ever noticed how our mind often works independently from us? How it can encourage or discourage us if it wants? How it can make us see things that aren't there, just by telling us that they are? It's time you regain control of your mind and tell it what to do for a change. You might think you are prepared for the worst - prepare your mind for it too. Exult in your success, but be wary of the future.

As you embark on another venture, I wish you success after success, so that there isn't enough time for depression to take over. Bon Voyage!

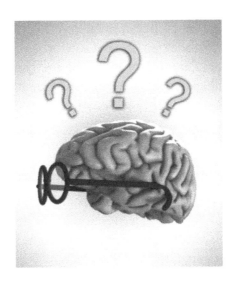

Chapter Ten:
Do You Know What Metaphor
You are Using?

"The logic of the emotional mind is *associative;* it takes
elements that symbolize a reality, or trigger a memory
of it, to be the same as that reality. That is why similes,
metaphors and images speak directly to the emotional
mind... If the emotional mind follows this logic and it's
rules, with one element standing for another, things need
not necessarily be defined by their objective identity:
what matters is how they are *perceived;* things are as they
seem... Indeed, in emotional life, identities can be like a
hologram in the sense that a single part evokes a whole."

- Daniel Goleman.

Whether you realize it or not, you have a metaphor you use to filter the experience of life through. I would add that most people are not aware of the metaphors they use. Once you understand how much our metaphors influence our experiences, though, you may find yourself taking far more interest.

One client of mine said, *"It's (dealing with his ADD symptoms) like fighting a war against a superior army!"* Take a moment and think about that statement. Notice what images come to mind, and what physical sensations you feel when you imagine fighting a war against a superior army. In the absence of any symptoms, that thought alone can be enough to trigger a stress response.

Now, imagine that my client used a different metaphor. Think about how differently he might experience his ADD with a metaphor of *"It's like raising a child to adulthood from infancy!"* When you think of this metaphor, does it create radically different images and feelings?

Is raising a child from infancy stressful? At times, very stressful. However, the underlying feeling of the experience you are having is one of love and commitment. It changes everything.

My client, while having used this metaphor many times throughout his life, wasn't aware of how deeply it was impacting him until I brought it to his attention. Once he had contrasted it with "softer" and more user-friendly metaphors, he was more than ready to drop his "war" processing.

How do you "drop" a metaphor, and adopt a different one? It's actually amazingly simple. First, become aware of the metaphors you are currently using. This can be as simple as paying more attention to how you talk about the various aspects of your life. However, a much faster way is to simply write down "ADD is like_____" or "Dealing with my ADHD symptoms is like_____".

While you will certainly benefit from looking at your ADD/ADHD specific metaphors, you'll also want to pay attention to the more global metaphors you use. "Life is like_____" is a global metaphor; it isn't looking at any particular context, its examining life in general.

My experience has been that in the areas of life where people are doing well, they almost always have supportive metaphors. Conversely, in the areas where they are challenged, their metaphors are less than useful.

Once you have identified a metaphor that is not something you would desire to pass on to your loved ones, begin to ask *"How would I like to think about this instead?"* Someone who is an artist, for example, might benefit from *"ADHD is like an oil painting."* Now, I have no idea what that means... I'm not an artist, but an artist, having a rich and textured understanding of how an oil painting is done, might understand that on levels that might very well prove to be therapeutic.

We are not born with "metaphors"; we unconsciously adopt and incorporate them as a way of understanding the world we live in. Ditch your old ones and pick up a few bright and shiny ones; it's like changing your jeans... when the pair you have on don't feel right, you keep trying new ones until you find a pair that feels good. Ooops... I think that was a metaphor ;)

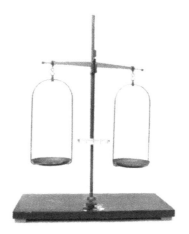

Chapter Eleven:
Both Are True, But Only One Is Useful

"Luck is a matter of preparation meeting opportunity."

- Oprah Winfrey.

One sunny morning two women wake up and get ready to head down stairs to make coffee. They are neighbors and live next to one another. On this particular morning, they both slip at the top of the stairs, and strangely, they both fall to the bottom of the stairs and slightly sprain their right wrists.

The first woman gets up, grabs her wrist and shouts, *"Damn! That's just how my luck goes; why should I be surprised, though? This kind of thing ALWAYS happens to me. This is going to be a bad day!"*

The other woman gets up, grabs the sprained wrist and gratefully says, *"Wheeww... that was close; I lucked out there! That could have been really bad. I could have broken by back, or even my neck, I'm fortunate. It will be hard to have a bad day after getting so lucky first thing in the morning!"*

You are probably way ahead of me. The only thing that that's "true" or a fact about both of these situations, is that they fell and sprained their wrists.

The assessment of both of these women is something they created... and opinion about what happened. They are both "right"; they are "right" in that once they have created, and then accepted their own assessment of what happened, it will set the direction for what they experience from that point on.

We are all entitled to our own opinion, but when we start to look more closely at how the opinion we create affects us, we often find that our opinion about something is more troubling than the situation itself.

The first woman will now be even more convinced than before that she has "bad luck". The second woman has yet another piece of "evidence" that she has always been a lucky woman. Because of her assessment, she will likely have a joyful day, telling others of how fortunate she had been that morning when she avoided a potentially catastrophic outcome.

If you have ADD and have just lost your third set of car keys in 6 months, you have a choice. You can focus on how, once again, you have "proof" of how ineffective your brain is or you can take a look at the things you have remembered in the last couple of days (which I can assure you will significantly outnumber the things you have lost) and feel thankful for the fact that you are able to keep track of so many things and, overall, lose very few things in the course of a year.

The choice is yours... choose as you wish. One choice will make you feel better; one will make you feel worse. Is it really that simple? Yes.

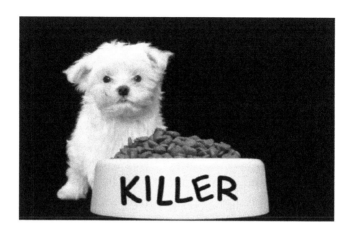

Chapter Twelve:
Choose Your Mate, Choose Your Fate

"The marriage state, with or without the affection suitable to it, is the most perfect image of Heaven and Hell we are capable of receiving in this life."

- Richard Steele, *The Spectator.*

Do you believe in the fact that things are preordained? Do you agree that if something has to happen it will happen, and that you were born on earth with a well-charted out plan of living, with a purpose that you were supposed to fulfill? In short, do you believe in "Fate"? I know many who do; ADD/ADHD and non-ADD/ADHD alike. I have nothing against fate, but I do have something against the effect it can have on people who believe in it too rigidly.

Rigid belief in fate is not good, for when things go in your favor you are prone to thinking that it's because of fate and if things go wrong, you believe it's been fated and there's little you can do to solve it. This is the reason I am a little wary of ADD/ADHD patients who unequivocally believe in the pre-ordainment of events in their life. They may approach physicians and other specialists to get help with their disorder, but internally they are convinced of the fact that they were fated to live through life with ADD/ADHD.

They come with a rigid mindset that can hinder progress. Why am I harping on about rigid belief in fate? Belief in fate by itself is not the problem; but one should believe in its flexibility and that they can change their fate by their actions, words and deeds.

Do you know of one very important component of your ADD/ADHD life? Your spouse. You have a choice when you decide to look for prospective mates, you can choose to set guidelines for fate to follow or believe in its indisputable power and jump blindly into marriage without analyzing whether the person you've married is capable of handling you at your worst.

Your partner will be one person you'll have to interact with day and night and who will (or rather should) stick by you through thick and thin. Your choice can make or mar your life. I have witnessed umpteen numbers of cases where the spouse cannot cope with the "challenges" of having an ADD/ADHD partner. It is not difficult to fall for someone with ADD/ADHD. They are creative, innovative and original, but to live through life with them requires that you be made of stronger stuff.

I am no marriage counselor, nor do I think I can take the liberty of telling you whom to marry; your parent I sure am not. Love has a curious way of just happening, but these are some practical observations you can make and actions you can take to ensure that the person you marry will accept you for what you are and be able to withstand the stress that can arise out of having to deal with ADD/ADHD behavior.

Come clean and let the person who's interested in you, or whom you wish to marry, know that you have ADD/ADHD. An honest approach in the beginning can save a lot of frustration, headache and heartache later on. The person might turn tail and run or may appreciate your honesty and be prepared for what is to come after marriage; either way you ensure that peace prevails.

Ask them if they understand the disorder and its gravity and whether they can live with it. Someone who gets irritated fast or tends to be intolerant of the idiosyncrasies that you know you have because of your ADD/ADHD, has poor scope of withstanding your behavior unless they decide to become more tolerant of it. For instance, some people hate forgetfulness and absentmindedness in others, but it's something ADD/ADHD people can do little about. This might go on to become a point of constant friction. So keep your eyes open and sieve the tolerant from the intolerant.

They should be willing to help. Having a partner who recognizes your condition and is willing to help you overcome your symptoms is a definite plus.

That said, having all the above qualities does not mean that you go for a spouse who will be a doormat, bearing with you as you go through your ADD/ADHD. Your domestic world would go for a toss in that case! Look for someone who's assertive and will set limits; that can help you through your symptoms kindly, but firmly. He or she should be able to look at you and see a normal spouse and be ready to do things couples normally do: *"you have to do the dishes tonight"* or *"you make breakfast tomorrow,"* for example.

All said and done, remember that your spouse is not the only one entering into this marriage; you are too. There will be things you'll have to do to make it work and you'd better be ready for them.

Go ahead, your fate awaits you.

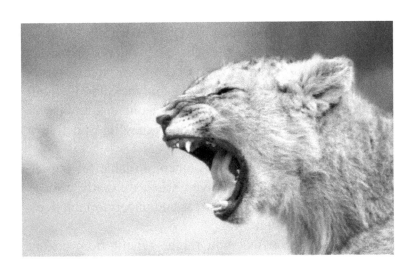

Chapter Thirteen:
Learn to Say "No" and Then Say It!

"The art of leadership is saying no, not saying yes. It is very easy to say yes."

- Tony Blair.

Most of us find it relatively easy to say "no" in an email message, or perhaps on the telephone, but when it comes to saying "no" face to face, well, that's a different story for many. We were taught to be polite, and not to do things others will find offensive.

Unfortunately, many of us have associated telling someone "no" with rejection, and since we find being rejected so painful, we strive to save others - and ourselves - the pain of hearing that awful two letter word.

An insurance salesman I know once told me that he always knew he had a sale waiting for him when he saw a sign on someone's door that read "No Solicitors". When I asked why, he said, "People who can't say no, and know they can't, find the only way to keep from buying everything that is offered to them is to avoid the offer. If someone has no qualms about telling someone else to beat it, there's no need for a sign on the door; they'll just deliver a firm 'No!' and that's that."

By striving to avoid any uncomfortable feelings in the "now" by telling people yes, when we really want to say no, we create a LOT of stress and uncomfortable feelings for the near future.

One question that you might benefit from asking yourself is, *"If I say yes to this, what will I be saying no to?"* See, if I say yes to going to a movie at 2:00 pm, I've just said no to everything else I could have done during that time. When you really get this, it can be a very life changing concept.

Let me ask you to consider something else. Let's say you had been to the doctor to get some blood tests done, and were waiting to hear back from them to find out whether you had some serious illness.

If you had an appointment to go find out your test results, and someone asked you to help out at a church luncheon, would you have a hard time telling them no? Of course not. Because you are so clear about the importance of your appointment, telling them no is about as easy as saying hello.

If you make it a habit of keeping the importance of your time fast at hand, then you'll always be able to decline the request of someone else. After all, what they are asking for is a chunk of your time - your limited time.

It's also important to note that loading yourself up with tasks that you don't really want, or have the time to do, will add to your stress levels. Remember a stressed mind is a cloudy mind. Time is a limited commodity. If you have 5 pieces of gum, and 7 people ask *"Can I have one?"* no matter how much you feel like saying yes, you know it's just not possible. When you begin to understand the concept of time, you'll see that it's much like the gum.

Like anything else, you'll get better at saying no with practice. Start saying no more often. You can always change your mind and say yes later, but that's the easy part. Start developing your "no" muscles today and say "Yes!" to yourself.

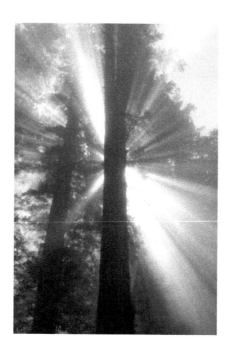

Chapter Fourteen:
Walk Towards the Light

"Until one is committed, there is hesitancy, the chance to draw back, always ineffectiveness. Concerning all acts of initiative (and creation), there is one elementary truth the ignorance of which kills countless ideas and splendid plans: that the moment one definitely commits oneself, the providence moves too. A whole stream of events issues from the decision, raising in one's favor all manner of unforeseen incidents, meetings and material assistance, which no man could have dreamt would have come his way."

- William Hutchinson Murray.

Everyone knows the feeling of getting up in the morning, knowing they have one or more tasks to do that they'd rather not. When you look at them on your list, or even in your mind, it's like they are a powerful spotlight shining right in your eyes.

The initial reaction is to put them off until later, and do the easier (and more enjoyable) tasks first. And, that's exactly what many people with ADD/ADHD do. Understandably, this adds to the stress later in the day; in the back of your mind, even while you are doing the simpler things, you know the "BIG" one is still waiting for you.

When the ADD/ADHD brain is stressed, it's like injecting a bowl of crystal clear water with jet black ink; everything becomes murky and cloudy. To the degree you can keep your stress level low, you can keep your mind clear, and a clear mind is a more efficient mind.

Some will argue *"Yes, but if I don't want to do it, it will be stressful no matter when I do it!"* To this I would say "Yes, it will probably be stressful no matter when you do it. However, when you do it early, the sense of relief that comes after it's done carries over into the rest of the day, and makes everything else seem incredibly pleasant by contrast."

When you have a task that's uncomfortable to think about - and is shining brightly back at you - walk towards it and tackle it first thing. When you "run" from it all day, it erodes your self-esteem and makes you feel like you are at the mercy of the world around you.

When you walk toward, confront and complete the thing you fear or find uncomfortable, your sense of power and self-confidence will sky rocket and you will flip things inside out; now you are directing your life, rather than being directed by your life.

Increasing your sense of control is perhaps more beneficial than what you actually get done when you "walk towards the light" and start your day with the things you used to put off until much later. Imagine the feeling of having all of the "nasty" stuff done by 9:00 am.

I'll tell you something else, something you already know; when you used to put things off until later in the day, each time a new "nasty" item popped onto your radar during the day, it seemed more overwhelming than it really was, only because you were already somewhat stressed about the "nasty" items you still hadn't done yet.

When you have cleared the slate first thing in the morning, you'll find your mind functioning much more clearly when the unexpected things show up later in the day. They just won't seem as intense when they aren't plopped down in the middle of several other "*I'd rather not do that!*" tasks.

Remember, walk towards the light. The brighter it shines, the more important it is to clear it from your list early in the day.

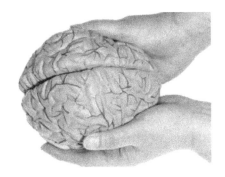

Chapter Fifteen:
Get Addicted to Things-Good Things

"I love making people laugh. It's an addiction and it's probably dysfunctional, but I am addicted to it and there's no greater pleasure for me than sitting in a theater and feeling a lot of people losing control of themselves."

- Jay Roach

ADHD is characterized by hyperactivity in many spheres of life. Coping with and soothing restlessness on a physical and mental plane drives many ADHD individuals to develop addictions. I have seen people fall into drug and alcohol abuse as they try to look for a way out of the mess in their brains and in their relationships.

Personally, I believe addiction is not bad if you are genetically or otherwise inclined towards it and can't seem to keep it at bay. If it helps you channel your frustration constructively, having an addiction might actually be a good thing. The question is not whether you have an addiction or not, the question is what is it that you are addicted to?

Most people with ADHD turn to alcohol to help them cope with their hyperactivity, some turn to marijuana, nicotine, caffeine and even sugar. You will surely find thousands of resources which tell you why these are not good, so it makes no sense for me to expound on it. What I would like to have you know is that these substances work, but only initially. They may help you "see things clearly" or help you focus on your tasks – substances like caffeine, nicotine and cocaine. But, instead of working as solutions to your problems, they bring with them addiction related problems, worsening your condition several fold.

However, just because you are addicted to something, doesn't mean you are a "bad" or "hopeless" human being. It was something your ADHD probably drove you to. That is not to say that just because you have ADHD, it is OK to be addicted. Absolutely not; but if you have an addictive behavior, you can channel your behavioral symptoms and frustrations into a "constructive addiction". What do I mean by that?

Think of good activities to do and write them down, by "good", I don't mean only morally or ethically good. Good means things that will benefit you without causing any harm to anyone else. After having written down what you consider to be good, select activities that you would like to do in order to channel your ADHD. Take for instance, exercising; if you want an activity to help you cope with your restlessness, hit the gym. Not only will you burn off the excess irritability over your frustrating symptoms, you'll also get an end product that will be so much better than what you would have gotten had you decided to use a bottle of alcohol or a shot of caffeine.

Find something that works for you, something that you like doing. You might be good at writing, write away your pains. Maintaining a diary helps a lot. Many things when put down on paper stop worrying us. Guilt, worries, and experiences can be penned down, so why not use it as a channel to help you cope with your ADHD?

If you are good at sports, then give sports a chance to help you fight your ADHD. Have you heard of people being addicted to their work? It is possible to use your work as a medium to forget the travails of being an ADHD person in a non-ADHD world. Not only will this help curb your restlessness, it will also influence your productivity and earn you brownie points with your boss.

Having a constructive addiction will not only help you, it will also raise your sense of self-esteem and give you a boost, the likes of which cannot be found by injecting amphetamines into your system. In fact, addictions of a destructive nature destroy not only your mental and physical faculties; they wreak havoc with your confidence, independence and sense of worth.

Searching for and zeroing in on "your addiction" is something that only you can do. It has to be an act that you love, something that you can lose yourself in, and feel happier and better after having done it.

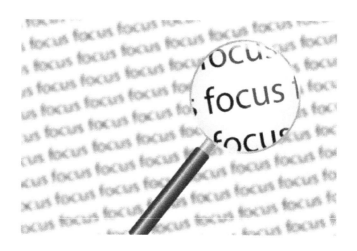

Chapter Sixteen:
Ben Franklin to the Rescue

"The secret of all victory lies in the organization of the non-obvious"

- Marcus Aurelius.

Benjamin Franklin is well known for saying "A place for everything and everything in its place." This is something that is foreign to many diagnosed with ADD/ADHD; when they are finished with something, it gets laid down wherever they might happen to be. When the item is needed again, they have to hunt and search, and after they finally find it, they repeat the cycle of use/lose (leave in the new location) and there it will remain until they find it on the next go around.

The best way to end the madness is so simple, that it's often overlooked.

Place things where they are most likely to be used or needed. To some, this may seem obvious, but to many with ADD/ADHD it's not. You won't be driving your car in the kitchen, so why put your keys there? Most people exit through the same door en route to their car 90% of the time; why not hang your car keys on a hook by the door? You can hang them there - and only there - each time you come in for the day, and pick them up on your way to the car. Nothing to guess about, worry about or look for, that's where you put them, and that's where they will be.

A dresser drawer is not a good place for someone with ADD/ADHD to put something. Why? Out of sight out of mind. If you are going to find a permanent place for a wallet, for example, make that somewhere out in the open; someplace where you can easily see the wallet when you look in that location.

One of my clients told me that he finally ended his nearly 25 year run of spending several minutes each day looking for his wallet by hanging it from a hook in a clear zip lock bag. Not only did he have it in the same place all of the time, but he could identify it from several feet away because he could see the wallet inside of the bag. He laughed, saying *I know it sounds crazy, but if it was in a black bag, I might go right past it, continuing my search for the wallet; unless I can see it, it's not there!*

This man stopped thinking about how silly his ritual might look or seem and, instead, started looking at what ritual would bring the most peace into his life.

Remember, when you are finished with something, put it back in its place - the ONLY place - and rest comfortably knowing where it will be the next time you need it. If it's there - and you know it - you don't have to think about it, and if you don't have to think about it, or struggle to remember where you might have used it last - and left it - then you have more of your attention available for other things. Automate, and then celebrate.

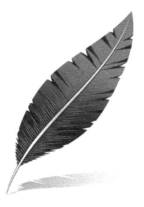

Chapter Seventeen:
Draw Sharp Lines

"Be yourself. Above all, let who you are, what you are, what you believe, shine through every sentence you write, every piece you finish."

- John Jakes.

When someone is first diagnosed with ADD or ADHD, they quickly start saying things like "us" or "we" when referring to people with the same diagnosis. It's like a Fraternity or Sorority they secretly take pride in belonging to. Identifying with others, solely on the basis of a diagnosis creates a belief that can lead to a dead end. Namely, the idea that what works for one person with ADD/ADHD will work for everyone.

In the previous chapter, I talked about a method for creating a place for everything. I also mentioned that you should put things close to where they will be used, and that's true... as long as it works for you!

If, for whatever reason, the organization method that works most effectively for you is something as counter-intuitive as putting things at the farthest point in the house from where you will use them, then that's what works for you.

Don't analyze it, don't run yourself crazy trying to figure it out, just realize that, for whatever reason, this method works better for you than the others, and continue to use it until something better is discovered.

Imagine yourself standing among tens of thousands of other people with ADD or ADHD. Then, imagine drawing sharp lines - a thick black circle - around yourself. Everything inside of the circle is unique to you, and everything inside everyone else's circle, unique to them. One person loves Mozart, another is wild about Nickleback, and still another is fond of B.B. King. Yes, they all have the same diagnosis, and they all like music, but buy them all the same CD for a birthday present and you've got problems.

You are unique; there is only one you. Let go of the idea that there is a "one size fits all" protocol and adopt what works for YOU. There are lots of solid ideas and methods in this book; some of them will change your life, some of them may do very little for you.

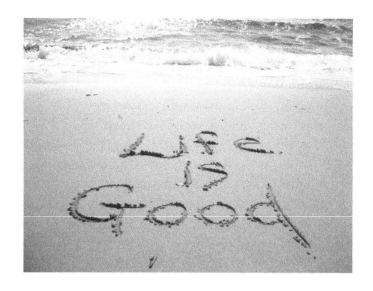

Chapter Eighteen:
Treating Your Social Life Like
it's Important

"Real answers need to be found in dialogue and interaction and, yes, our shared human condition. This means being open to one another instead of simply fighting to maintain a prescribed position."

- Malcolm Boyd.

"I just can't seem to get along with people." I've lost count of the number of times I've heard ADD/ADHD adults tell me that they are completely at a loss when it comes to social interactions. For successful interactions, one needs to possess certain social skills. If you've read Dale Carnegie's "How to Win Friends and

Influence People", you must have noticed the amount of emphasis he puts on good listening abilities. If you can listen, people will call you a good communicator.

Let's look at you. You have ADD/ADHD, reason enough to justify inattentiveness, hyperactivity and impulsiveness. These very characteristics in a person who does not have ADD/ADHD, and even in one who does, are completely undesirable. How does each of these affect your ability to interact with your friends or colleagues?

Imagine you are about to leave for work and your wife calls out that you have to visit an ailing relative, who's on her deathbed (just to make it more interesting) today at 4.00 pm in the hospital. What you hear is *"You have to visit Aunt Wilma today"* and the rest of it tunes out as your inattentiveness takes over. You make your way to the hospital at 6.00 pm after you leave your office. But wait; the visiting hours were from 4.00-6.00 and you are forbidden entry. Poor Aunt Wilma passes away peacefully in her sleep that night.

This instance of your inattentiveness was in a domestic setting, but it can take you over anywhere, anytime, while you are conversing with your boss, your friend, your relative, your kid or your dog. To the person conversing with you, it may seem as though you couldn't care less.

Inattentiveness leads to regret and strained relationships. Work towards overcoming it. It helps to keep a tab on your thinking when you are conversing with someone else. As soon as you catch yourself drifting, give yourself a mental whack and bring yourself back to the conversation. If you realize that you might have missed something during the course of the conversation, do not hesitate to ask for a repetition, it will save you and the other person a lot of misunderstanding.

You are in a meeting and your ADHD is acting up. You just can't sit still; you feel the need to release the hyperactive-ness building up inside you. Enclosed spaces or social events where you are supposed to stay put in one place might tax your patience, but that is one of the several social graces you are expected to have. Inability to do so will give people an impression of disinterest, which I am sure you don't want to portray.

The impulsive behavior of ADD/ADHD persons manifests itself in conversations too. Constantly interrupting the person who is talking is something ADHD individuals can't help doing. Talking non-stop and speaking out whatever comes to your mind all hint to your ADHD induced impulsiveness. Not only will the person get irritated and lose interest in what you wish to say, but you might also end up saying something you regret because of your impulsiveness. As I said before, people like good listeners, if you are going to be doing all the talking; your likeability will be highly questionable.

No matter how tedious it may sound, making social contact with people is a very important part of our lives. You cannot hide yourself behind the curtain of ADHD/ADD, because the curtain is transparent. Huh? You do know, I suppose, that ADHD and ADD are not visible, in-your-face disorders. Someone conversing with you will not know that your inattentive, impulsive or hyperactive behavior can be blamed on to your ADD/ADHD. What they will see is only you, without the curtain that you imagine is there, standing aloof from the crowd.

Make the effort to reach out and learn the social skills. Get in touch with friends, schedule a time and place to meet them and keep to the schedule. Connect with people; you need them in your life. Nobody travels alone and the journey will never be weary if conversation and laughter flows freely. Here's to a social you!

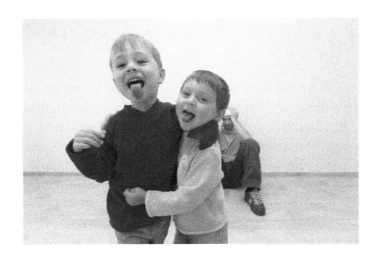

Chapter Nineteen:
Loosen Up and Be Willing to Get Goofy!

"What monstrous absurdities and paradoxes have resisted whole batteries of serious arguments, and then crumbled swiftly into dust before the ringing death-knell of a laugh!"

- Agnes Repplier

"*Mirror, mirror on the wall! Who's the goofiest of them all?*" Clap your hands, laugh out loud, and prove to the mirror that you are the clown. Go to parties and dance to all songs, laugh at yourself if you go wrong.

"*Hey! What's with the rhymes?*" you ask. Nothing, I am just feeling a bit goofy. Have you ever laughed hard and loud at yourself? Have you gone wrong sometime, somewhere and had people laugh at you, but couldn't hear their laughter, not because you were embarrassed, but because you were laughing the loudest?

It is a good feeling, this goofiness. It can inject humor in the most serious of situations and help you get over your embarrassment when you make a mistake. Laughter is a gift and to be able to laugh and make others laugh can give immeasurable joy. If you believe any of the various sayings about laughter; "laughter is the best medicine" or "laugh and the world laughs with you" and so on and so forth, you should consider yourself blessed indeed that you have many more reasons to laugh than a non-ADD/ADHD person.

"How does my ADD/ADHD have anything to do with how much I laugh?" If you can't improve a situation, learn to make the best of it. You've got to live with your ADD/ADHD and you will keep committing mistakes that people with ADD/ADHD are wont to do. You'll keep forgetting things, which in itself can be a source of innumerable funny cases. You'll keep shooting impulsive things from your mouth; keep tuning out every five minutes and keep mishearing things. I am not making fun of your disorder; just gently suggesting that you change your view of your situation. Stop being defensive and avoiding social contact just because you feel you'll be laughed at.

Laughter has a way of taking the edge off insults aimed at you. It can help dissipate unsavory confrontations. If you make a mistake, you might be laughed at, in which case you should join in the laughter! Or you might be reprimanded - admit your mistake and be ready to take the blame cheerfully - others will be more willing to forgive you.

Here are some pointers which might help you give up feeling sorry for yourself and take on a more humorous approach to life and your ADD/ADHD:

1. **Recognize when your ADD/ADHD is acting up:** Be aware of your actions and recognize which slips can be attributed to ADD/ADHD and which can't.

2. **Practice your laugh:** When you do something silly, like end up in the bathroom when you were heading for the living room, because you forgot where you were going…laugh your head off at yourself! Practice the laugh and you'll perfect it in time.

3. **Don't isolate yourself:** Your fear of criticism and ridicule is no reason to shut yourself out of social interactions. You'll learn to cope in time. Learn to laugh off the teasing; people will like you all the more.

4. **Loosen up:** Don't carry an image of yourself with you. Don't be rigid and scared to let down your guard. Let life take you where it wants in your social interactions… Let go!

5. **Be forgetful:** Forgetfulness might be a characteristic of ADD/ADHD but it is surprising how many ADD/ADHD people refuse to forget an incident in which they feel they've been slighted. Don't let past experiences hinder your future growth.

Get in touch with old friends and behave as if you haven't a care in the world. People who care for you will not be exceedingly judgmental of your actions, or "misactions". Practice your humor in front of them first, if you think your ADD/ADHD has rendered it rusty.

Given time, you'll learn to laugh at yourself, not unlike Naseeruddin Hodja of Turkey, the witty, satirical character of the 13th century. People were jealous of him not only because he was the sultan's favorite, but more so because he could laugh at himself. So drop those shackles you've chained around yourself, loosen up and get goofy!

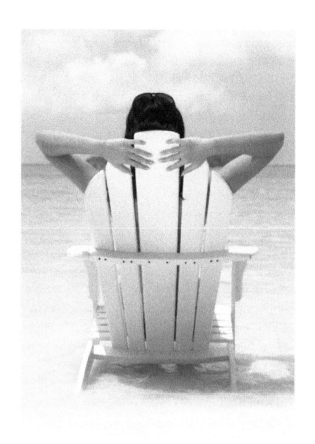

Chapter Twenty:
Talk to Yourself

"The essence of strategy is choosing what not to do."

- Michael Porter.

Technology today offers the ability to do things that just a few years ago would have seemed ridiculous. No longer do we have to use miles of audio "reel to reel" tape for a recording. Now, for less than $40 we can purchase a digital voice recorder that is about half the size of a pack of cigarettes that will hold hours of recordings. A device such as this can make your life much easier.

Because of its small size, carrying a digital voice recorder is a cinch; shirt or jacket pockets are ideal. With this "extra brain" on hand, any thought that crosses your mind can be captured easily and effortlessly. Writing your thoughts down is great; being able to actually look at them on paper can offer a distinct advantage.

However, there are times when stopping to write an idea down on paper just isn't feasible. When you are driving, outside doing yard work or on a morning walk, it's much easier to click the "record" button and talk, than it is to carry a notepad and pen, and then stop to write down what you want to remember.

If you've ever had a brilliant idea, but a few days later couldn't remember the idea - just that you had thought of one a few days ago - then you know how frustrating it can be when you let something escape your consciousness and long term memory. Don't trust your memory. Capture the thoughts that you think you'd like to have access to later.

After you get home, or back to the office, take the ideas you recorded and transcribe them; write them down in a notebook or "to do" list you can refer to. Because so much of information processing by our brain is in the visual mode, writing it down can assist you in thinking about what you recorded with even greater clarity.

Just in case you are thinking *"using a digital recorder is a crutch; I ought to be able to remember on my own,"* I ask you this: Is the doctor who is using an antibiotic to treat your infection using a "crutch"? I mean, after all, if he was really good, couldn't he just use natural substances like the Native American Indians did?

Use whatever is available to make it easier for you to be more effective and productive. To do anything less is to do yourself, and those around you, a huge disservice.

Once you have made carrying a digital recorder a habit, you'll never want to be without one again. Oh, did I mention that when you first get one, you should keep it in the same place at the end of the day? Just checking.

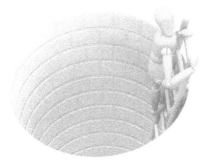

Chapter Twenty One:
Fail and Succeed

"Every person who wins in any undertaking must be willing to cut all sources of retreat. Only by doing so can one be sure of maintaining that state of mind known as a burning desire to win - essential to success."

- Napoleon Hill.

Do you sometimes catch yourself day dreaming when you need to be focusing on the task at hand? My bet is that the more you try to focus, the more you "slip" into day dreaming. This frustrating cycle can all but wear you down.

Fortunately, there's something you can do; something that seems insane, backwards and highly unlikely to work. That's exactly why most people rarely discover this one on their own.

Do you remember the last time someone was taking your picture and they said "smile"? More often than not, when you see the pictures that were taken while you were putting a smile on your face at request, it looks, well... less than genuine. When we take a behavior that has been occurring automatically and unconsciously, and then try to create it on cue, we almost always find the process to be difficult at best.

Ask someone who gets embarrassed when they meet someone of the opposite sex to do so on demand, beginning a few minutes before they are to meet the person, and you're likely to be met with "I can't!"

Even if they are able to succeed at getting a little bit embarrassed, they'll find it to be a weaker version, and most importantly, they'll have shifted "embarrassment" from something that happens to them, to something over which they have more conscious control. Either way, they win.

Watch what happens the next time you are day dreaming and, after catching yourself, you give the self-command to day dream even deeper, longer or more clearly. You'll probably fail, and in failing, you find that the failure is identified by the recognition that you are more focused and in the present moment - the opposite of day dreaming.

Sound strange? It should, it's truly something that very few people have ever heard or thought about. On one level it makes no sense, and yet, on another level, it makes perfect sense.

How else can you use this to help with ADD/ADHD? The next time you are worrying excessively about something, make an appointment to worry. That's right; put it on your schedule: Tonight from 7:00 - 7:30 I'll go to a quiet room and worry. You can probably already guess what will happen. You'll find yourself thinking about everything but what you had been worrying about earlier.

Take some time to identify the behaviors, thoughts and feelings that have been troubling and have also occurred automatically. Next, decide to do this behavior on cue; at a particular time or place. By putting this previously unconscious and automatic behavior into the framework of intentional and conscious effort, you'll be jamming the very structure that had allowed it to function so smoothly.

Sometimes I'll have someone say *"I don't think that will work, that sounds crazy!"* I'll ask them, *"Has the way you've been trying ever worked?"* *"No,"* they'll reply. *"And yet you continue?"* I ask with a grin. *"What can be any crazier than that?"* Most will say, *"You're right. What do I have to lose?"*

The truth is you have absolutely nothing to lose from employing this method, and everything to gain, so go ahead and enjoy succeeding by failing.

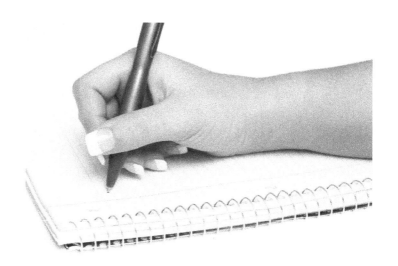

Chapter Twenty Two:
The Notebook Trick for
Remembering More

"So when you are listening to somebody, completely, attentively, then you are listening not only to the words, but also to the feeling of what is being conveyed, to the whole of it, not part of it."

- Jiddu Krisnamurti.

If you've ever lost your keys, your wallet, your purse, or forgotten all about that important appointment, you're about to learn something that has the potential to transform your life in ways you can't even imagine.

Have you ever stopped to wonder why you can so easily forget where you put the mail after you walked in the house? Most of the time, it comes down to not being conscious of putting the mail down while you were putting it down.

Your mind had already jumped several steps ahead, and when you placed the mail on the table (or wherever it was you put it) it simply did not break through your awareness.

The fastest way I know of to notice more of what you're doing, while you're doing it, is to start keeping a journal. Each night, before going to bed, write down as much of what you can remember about your day; where you went, who you talked to and what you did.

At first, you'll probably find that you don't remember quite everything. When you realize that you can't recall much of your day, and know that you'll be writing things down again the next night, you'll naturally find yourself paying more attention to the things you are doing, while you are doing them.

As you begin paying closer attention, you'll find that you are able to remember - with great detail - the events of the day. This leads to less forgetting and that leads to less stress.

The human brain loves rewards, and each time you are able to recall something, the brain will process it like a prize or reward it has earned. This "end of the day" journal is a selfre-enforcing method.

The more successful you are; the more successful will you want to be. The better you get; the better you will get and the more attention you'll be devoting to each task of the day.

There's another advantage of this technique. When you start recording each day, you begin noticing the overall quality and effectiveness of each day.

It's one thing to waste half the day without really knowing or thinking about it, but when you are actually looking at what you have - or have not - accomplished for several days running, it has a way of getting you to want to get more out of life than you have been.

What more could you want for the price of a notebook and ballpoint pen? The simple act of recording each day improves both your memory and your outlook, helping you focus more clearly on your life's purpose. If you don't know your life's purpose yet, it will help you recognize that too.

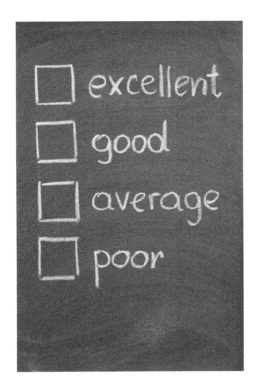

Chapter Twenty Three:
How an "F" Equals an "A"

"The greatest mistake you can make in life is to
continually fear you will make one."

- Elbert Hubbard.

All I can say about what I'm about to share with you
is "WOW!" It's new, and best of all - it works; I've used

it myself, and the difference in recall, later on (after using this method) is nothing short of amazing.

Let's say you wanted to get your license to sell insurance in your state of residence. Traditionally, people will gather all of the study guides available on the subject and then spend weeks pouring over page after page of mind-boggling material. But when using this method to learn, just how much of the information is retained? Several studies indicate that recall is sad - really sad - when most people are tested again a few weeks later.

Obviously, in some cases this method may prove to be effective, however, there is an alternative to spending weeks studying.

So, what is this new method? Plan to take the test twice. Forget about studying for the first one; just go take it and do the best you can, with no expectation of any particular grade - or of passing.

The results of a study published in the Journal of Experimental Psychology: *Learning, Memory and Cognition*, conducted at the University of California (Los Angeles) provide strong evidence that taking a test and guessing at the answers will not only allow you to learn more easily, but also to hang onto what you learn a heck of a lot longer than the now antiquated method of preparing for a test by "learning it all" beforehand.

By guessing at the answers - and getting many of them wrong - your mind will be primed to learn more easily and quickly recall the right answer when you do your actual studying before taking the "real" test.

How much of a difference does this make? In terms of making the information "easier" to learn, studies have found the increase to be about 10%.

When it comes to being able to recall the information two weeks later, the difference is even more striking: students who pre-tested remembered 60% of the material two weeks later, compared to the students who did not pre-test and were only able to recall 40% of what they had previously learned.

Is this just for academic work or test taking? No, no, no!

How many times a week do you run to the computer to look for the answer to something that pops into your head? Instead of simply typing the keywords into the search engine and waiting for the answer, take a few moments to come up with the answer on your own.

Give it your best shot; think about it for a minute and guess the answer, trying to get as close as you can. This simple method will substantially increase your recall. Rather than finding the answer and then having to say *"Oh, darn it... I can't remember... I just looked it up the other day!"* when talking to someone else, you will likely find the answer much closer to the "front" of your mind.

Where else can you use this to ease the previous challenges of ADD/ADHD?

Not everything you remember has to be highly valued information. Maybe you go to a concert, and would just like to be able to remember the first 5 songs your favorite band plays so you can tell your friends later.

Before you go, just guess; write down what you think the first 5 songs will be. Each time you use this method, you'll be more likely to use it again, and again, and again. Use it, have fun, and enjoy remembering things better and longer.

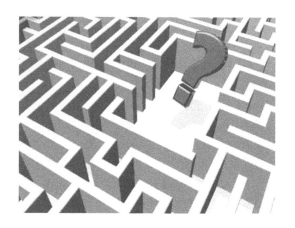

Chapter Twenty Four:
Be Able to Identify What You Want
- With Precision

"Imagination is as vital to any advance in science as learning and precision are essential for starting points."

- Percival Lowe.

A patient of mine told this story: *"Thirty four years ago, when I was in the second grade I was diagnosed with attention deficit disorder and was prescribed Ritalin to 'help' me out. Now what were they helping me out with? My teachers used to say I spent too much time 'daydreaming' and 'talking' and that it was going to make it hard for me to accomplish anything if I couldn't get those things under control. I can't tell you how ironic it is to be doing those two things for a living now. As a writer and professional speaker, that's what I do; I get to daydream and talk!"*

This man had finally aligned himself with the way his brain naturally preferred to function, and is now living a life he thought to be impossible at one time.

Daydreaming or letting your mind run wild is the first step in knowing what you want to do, in making that discovery of what you do best, of what makes you feel alive. Oliver Wendall Holmes said *"Most will go to their graves with the music still in them."* There are few things I can think of that are as sad as the thought of going to my grave never having played the music that's in me.

Most people, when they really stop and think about it, have a rough idea of what they'd really like to do, feel or experience. And I say rough idea, because when you ask them for any specific details, they get this blank look on their face. Sometimes people will tell me, *"I just want to feel happy again"* and yet, when I ask them, *"How will you know when you feel that way? If you went to bed tonight, and as you slept a miracle occurred, and when you woke up you had been transformed into a happy person.... how would you know?"*

I've never had someone launch into the explanation, describing in detail how they would know, or what it would feel like...never. For most people, their eyes will glaze over and they'll stare off into wonderland, and then it's usually at least 5 - 10 minutes before they're able to accurately describe how they would know.

I might add that before they begin to tell me what they would feel like if they were happy, I get this big list of what they *wouldn't* feel like if they were happy. Knowing what you won't feel is a long way from knowing what you WILL feel.

Imagine that I have severely burned my arm, and I call the emergency room. I tell them *"I'm worried about my arm."* When they ask me to describe what's wrong, I say *"Well, it doesn't have a dull ache, it doesn't have a stabbing type pain, and it doesn't feel itchy!"*

Do they have any idea whatsoever what my arm DOES feel like? Of course not. Our brains need input about what we DO want. When you create a blueprint for your brain, showing it exactly what you DO want, you'll be amazed at the speed that you'll start moving towards those things, accomplishments or feelings.

How specific do you have to be? I don't think you can be too specific. The more detail you can provide, the more accurately your brain can start sorting and looking for experiences that will match, and that will become re-sources for you.

Do you want a new car? What model? Okay a new mustang. What color? What wheels do you want? How about the interior, what color and options do you want? Does it come with more than one size of motor? Which one do you want?

You want to be confident? How will you know when you are? What images will you have in your mind? What kinds of things will you say to yourself? What will your posture be like when you feel confident? Where do you notice your breathing when you feel this way? What are the particular facial expressions and hand gestures that go along with feeling confident? What clothes do you wear when you feel really confident? Is there any particular jewelry that you might wear?

This is just a brief example of the kind of specificity I'm talking about. You can go through the rest of your life talking about a new car and confidence, but if you don't provide your mind with the details, you'll often wind up creating or feeling something that's very different from what you really want.

It might help if you think about this by framing it as creating the environment in which your brain can learn most effectively. Because that's really what you're doing... you're teaching your brain *"Hey this is what I want!"* What you get back is really a statement about your effectiveness as a teacher. Researchers know that learning literally changes the brain; every time we learn something new it actually alters our brain structure. One of the most important stages of learning is the concept of pre-exposure.(You do remember Pre-exposure, don't you?) Pre-exposure primes our brain; it creates a foundation that we can then build connections on. The better the background, the faster the learning will occur.

Think of describing what you want in detail as a form of pre-exposure for your brain. This will help you learn even more about what you want, because the more you can describe and notice, the more you will be able to describe and notice.

The next time you walk by a tree, stop and pick off a leaf. Then for perhaps the first time in your life, look at it in detail. Turn it over, and feel how the texture differs from one side to the other. Does it have a smell? Notice all of the intricate details of the little lines on the leaf. If you really take the time to do this, you won't believe how much is there that you have never appreciated before. But here's what I want you to discover, as you are looking at this leaf; each time you notice something new, you are able to then see even more, or something that exists another level down. This same thing happens when you begin describing in detail the kinds of feelings you want to experience.

The more you can describe what your body is experiencing when you're feeling good, the more you become aware of the sensations in your body, and this is a critical step in being able to alter your feelings, and to notice that when you make changes in your physiology, it also changes how clearly and precisely you think. So feel free to use this principle of being incredibly precise about what you want.

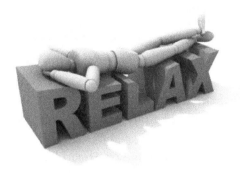

Chapter Twenty Five:
What You Do Today, is Easier to Do To-morrow

"Good habits, once established are just as hard to break as are bad habits"

- Robert Puller.

When you were first learning to tie your shoes, you developed the habit of putting one of your shoes on first. Maybe it's the right one, or it might be the left. Just start to observe which shoe you put on first, because after you have acknowledged which one it is, you'll have the chance to find out how bizarre and uncomfortable it can feel to switch things up, and put the other one on first.

Why is this huge deal? It's a huge deal because it shows us how something as simple as which shoe we put on first can become neurologically etched for comfort and familiarity.

But here's the thrilling part; if you'll just permit yourself to be comfortable about being uncomfortable for a very short period of time, you'll soon find that you're just as comfortable putting on the opposite shoe as the one you had been putting on first. Our nervous system is so malleable, that given enough time and corroboration, we can retrain ourselves to make any actions or feeling as natural as the one we are replacing.

Look, some people have practiced feeling bad for 45 years and falsely think that it would be a waste of time to try, as they say, to "teach an old dog new tricks." But let me ask you, do you think it took that person 45 years to be able to feel lousy all the time, or do you think they mastered it swiftly, and then just repeated it over and over, getting faster at being able to access this un-resourceful state of being? The fact is, humans are learning machines, and we learn much faster than we think, and not just as children, but at all ages.

I don't care if you've had 94 years of experience accessing un-resourceful states of mind, the instant *you decide to do something different*, and then *begin to do something different*, you are making it easier to do the next day, and the next, and so on.

As you look forward, out to future months and years, what would you like to be doing - habitually - in 5 years, 10 years and beyond? Whatever it is, chances are very good indeed, that if you simply begin now, and repeat again each new day, before you know it, you will have replaced the old ADD/ADHD associated behaviors with the new, different, and considerably more productive ones. Enjoy!

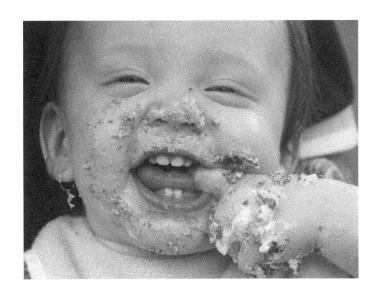

Chapter Twenty Six:
Do Not "Take" Until You Are
Prepared to "Replace"

"First say to yourself what you would be; and then do what you have to do."

- Epictetus.

You've probably watched one of the big forest fires that are sporadically shown on the news, where thousands of acres burn leaving nothing but the barren ground beneath the once lush landscape. But a short time later the naked land will have changed into a beautiful and picturesque backdrop once again.

Our mind works in a comparable way. Have you ever noticed what happens to many smokers when they finally quit smoking? They start eating and snacking at the times they used to smoke, and often times will gain a substantial quantity of weight.

Of course, I understand that some of that has to do with the fact that nicotine has been shown to be somewhat of an appetite suppressant. However, I also know that we are patterned behaviorally.

If your mind and body has been used to walking in and out of your office 15 times before ever getting started on your work for the day, there will be a great desire to continue in using this same pattern... it's familiar

But you know this is going to happen, so you might as well make a conscious selection about what the substitute pattern is going to be. Just realize that when you're going to create an empty space, by "quitting" some previous behavior or less than useful cognitive course of action, you'll want to come up with the replacement first. Otherwise, that "empty spot" won't be empty for long.

You'll either have enjoyed the fulfillment of being the one to decide what goes in its place, or, you'll discover that something has already taken it.

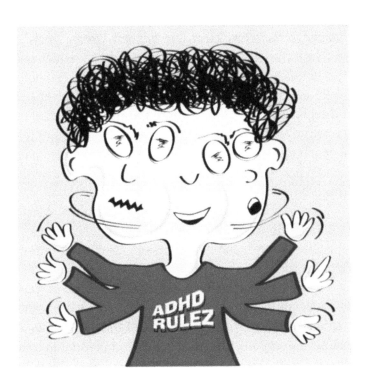

Chapter Twenty Seven:
Be Careful with Your ADD/ADHD Goals

"Paradoxically though it may seem, it is none the less true that life imitates art far more than art imitates life."

- Oscar Wilde.

I'll bet you've heard about the famous study on goals conducted at Yale many years ago.

In this study - a study that was initiated in 1953 - researchers surveyed those who were graduating from Yale. After the survey the researchers found that only 3% of the graduating seniors had clear and explicit written goals. 20 years later it was discovered that the 3% that had written goals had accumulated more wealth than the other 97% combined.

Remarkable right? The *story* is remarkable, but you see, there's one BIG problem with the story: it's a lie. Yale University Research Associate, Beverly Waters completed a far-reaching search, digging through Yale records and archives. What was her conclusion? The study is an urban myth - it NEVER HAPPENED.

I have to admit, on my personal development path I bought hook, line and sinker into this compelling story. So did just about everyone else that was striving to improve their lot in life.

Let me make one thing clear: Goals ARE powerful tools for accomplishing more than you would have without them, but *only* if you are able to avoid the deadly mistake that almost everyone makes, and we'll get to that in a moment.

First, though, take a moment to consider all of the things in your life that you *have* accomplished, things you are proud of, that you didn't have a goal about. As you begin to look at your life in detail, you'll see that some of your greatest accomplishments did not spring forth from a written goal - you just did what had to be done and accomplished them.

Next (and this can be a little depressing) think about all of the things you *did* set goals for, but that you never even came close to achieving. If you've been a "goal setter" for many years, don't think about this for too long, because this list, for most people, is longer than they would like.

Most people, when establishing their goal, focus on how they will feel, how happy, how rich, how content, how ecstatic - you name it - *after* they have accomplished their goal. They rationalize *"If I pick something very rewarding, something that will really be worth having <u>in the future</u>, I'll be able to endure anything I have to get there."* Almost everyone is overly optimistic about their capability to do things in the future. What they forget about, however, is that the future is only a concept, a thought, and that the only thing that ever truly exists is NOW, the present moment. Life is one present moment after the other from cradle to grave.

If the goal you pick is one that will *not* allow you to feel inspired, driven, excited, and invigorated in *every present moment* between right now and the achievement of your goal, then you have picked the wrong goal.

From now on, when you are about to write down a goal, ask *"How will having this goal impact my 'right nows'? Will having this goal cause me to wake up each day and feel excited to jump out of bed and get started?" "Will having this goal cause me to have to pry myself away from it each night to go to bed?"* If the answer is "Yes!" press on. If the answer is "No!" move on.

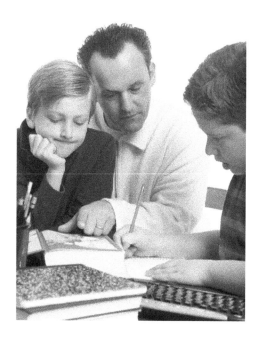

Chapter Twenty Eight:
Be an Advocate for Yourself

"I've learned you can make a mistake and the whole world doesn't end. I had to learn to allow myself to make a mistake without becoming defensive and unforgiving."

-Lisa Kudrow.

"But this is so simple, how could you possibly not do it?" "What! You forgot to get the file again! How many times do I need to remind you?" These are diluted versions of the kind of criticism you might face daily, if you are a

person with ADD/ADHD. Having to listen to people admonishing you day and night for something you just can't help can get frustrating. The frustration can manifest itself in various ways and when coupled with your ADD/ADHD symptoms, it can completely wear you out.

What most people do in response to criticism is get defensive and try to justify their point of view. ADD/ADHD individuals face so much criticism, that being defensive becomes a part of their life and a part of their communication with people. Real or imagined criticism can bring their defensiveness to the fore. When you are overly defensive, you lose a lot and gain nothing. You miss the other person's point of view, as you drown out their voice in trying to justify your actions, irrespective of whether that justification is warranted or not.

Defensiveness is good, up to a limit. It is a sort of protection against assumed or real threats. It has helped man enter the 21st century. If our bodies weren't defensive and didn't mount an immunologic response against every perceived or real pathogen that managed to gain entry, the human race would not be here to grace the new millennia or even the one before that. But emotional defensiveness is a different ball game altogether.

You can't be emotionally defensive all the time. You will miss out on opportunities, potential relationships and knowledge. How so?

Imagine you've gone for an interview and the employer says, "*OK. So you have ADHD?*" and you immediately launch into a half-an-hour long barrage about how you may have the disorder, but it is not severe enough to hinder your activities and how you do everything that someone who does not have ADHD can do, and so on and so forth. Now look back and tell me what the answer should have been. You could have simply answered "*Yes.*" Thereafter, you give him, or her, the choice to ask you what they wish to know about your abilities to cope with the disorder. By switching into a defensive mode as soon as you hear ADHD, you reaffirm his or her belief that you are hyperactive. There goes your prospective job down the drain.

Become an advocate for yourself. Have clear cut knowledge of who you are, how you are and what is it that you lack. Try to improve on the characteristics that you know are not desirable to have. If you can't, then go ahead and make peace with the fact that you can't and that it is a part of you.

Once you've learnt to relax around your shortcomings and accept them as a part of you, others' criticisms of those same characteristics will stop hurting you. Also, the next time you start feeling defensive in any situation, stop to analyze where the defensiveness is coming from. There might been a similar situation in the past when you have gotten hurt and are trying to emotionally protect yourself this time around. Did you overreact then? Was your response in excess to the provocation? Don't repeat that mistake again.

Sometimes, it's better to let your inattentiveness take over when you think you are being emotionally threatened, than to get defensive and worked up. Man uses (or, rather, overuses) a lot of mechanisms to combat emotional pain, whether real or presumed. Think alcohol, illicit drugs and un-prescribed, over-the-counter medications. Similarly, defensiveness is a rampantly used mode of self-protection. Cut down on your consumption of defensiveness and curb your impulses to jump at the person's neck at the slightest hint of criticism. When you begin to hear something you don't like, lean back and zip your mouth. Give the person three minutes to get back on line and if they refuse to do so, then shut them out. Ignorance is bliss.

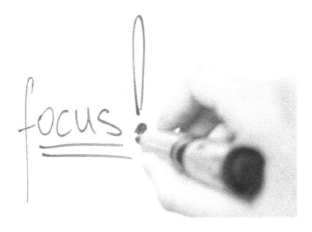

Chapter Twenty Nine:
Learn More About Learning

"Personally, I am always ready to learn, although I do not always like being taught."

- Winston Churchill.

If you want to learn - really learn - virtually anything in life, faster and more effectively than ever before, it's critical to understand the 5 Stages of Learning.

Many of the struggles that people have experienced with ADD/ADHD have involved the inability to learn and/ or remember as well as their non - ADD/ADHD peers. When you understand and incorporate the 5 Stages of Learning, you'll be surprised at how easy it was to reach this new and improved you, learning and remembering with ease.

Stage One: Pre-Exposure - By pre-viewing the material or information you wish to learn, it literally primes the neural networks of your brain, doing something akin to pre-heating the oven before you put the turkey in that you'll be having for dinner.

In text books, read the chapter headings and the summary a few hours (preferably the night) before you are going to read it in detail. The more you know that relates to the new material before you are introduced to it, the more quickly the information will be acquired.

Stage Two: Acquisition - In short, this is where the information you wish to learn is encountered. This may be the first time you read a text in detail, listen to a lecture or watch a video.

Once new information has been received through sensory input, additional synaptic connections take place, and your neurons are actually engaged in a process of communicating with one another. Prior knowledge of the subject (pre-exposure) determines how effective the acquisition stage will be.

Stage Three: Elaboration - This one means you need to expand on what you took in during acquisition. For example, you can tell me all about the steps involved in riding a bicycle and, on one level I can understand. However, until I have elaborated on that knowledge - and actually hopped on a bike - my learning will be far from complete.

Let's take another example. If you were learning to play say, Black Jack, or 21, for the first time, you might do well to begin reading about what cards to "hit" on, and which cards to "hold", but there is nothing more effective than playing with someone who already understands the game, long before you think you are ready. This real time feedback will do wonders.

Stage Four: Memory Formation - Ever crammed all night for a test - studying until daylight - and then rushing into class to take it? If so, you probably know that about 30 minutes after you have taken the test, you can barely remember what topic you were studying. The reason for this is fairly straight - forward; REM sleep is crucial if memory formation is to occur. Without sleep, you can just about forget about anything more than short-term memory.

Another significant factor in memory formation is the emotional intensity of the action. The stronger the emotion, the more lasting the memory. This is why, after years of marriage, many people have a very un-balanced perspective of their relationship. It's often easier to remember the arguments than the good times; "good" times are often fairly calm, but arguments generally have high-intensity emotions attached.

Stage Five: Functional Integration - You've no doubt heard the "Use it or lose it!" phrase on occasion. When it comes to learning and long-term memory this is certainly the case.

You can recall, perhaps, the overwhelming situation presented by so many things to keep track of when you first learned to drive. Now, chances are good that you don't consciously think of all of those driving behaviors that used to require your full and complete attention.

This is an example of functional integration. Sure, you had already learned something of value once you first got your license; you did "know" the information needed for the written test, and were able to demonstrate a working knowledge of the car itself, but after months or years of repetition, a more thorough kind of learning has taken place - functional integration.

By keeping the 5 Stages of Learning in mind, you can choose to begin, and successfully complete, any process of learning.

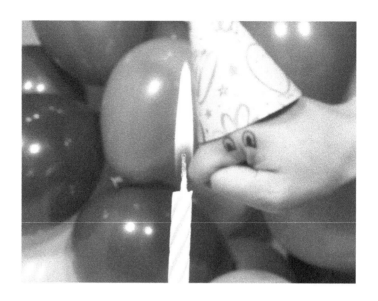

Chapter Thirty:
Design Your Environment to "Inflate" Rather Than "Deflate"

"You are a product of your environment. So choose the environment that will best develop you toward your objective. Analyze your life in terms of its environment. Are the things around you helping you toward success - or are they holding you back?"

-Richard Bach.

How long have you had your ADD/ADHD? If you had it as a kid, you will identify with what I have to say. Think back to your school days. I don't know how you remember those days. You might remember them with fondness, or perhaps you don't want to think of them at all, especially if school brought out the worst of your ADD.

School can be an example of a deflating environment, if yours wasn't very ADD/ADHD friendly. What do I mean by that? Your school life probably had a non-ADD/ADHD conducive environment; maybe it was designed in such a way as to provide maximum benefit to the maximum number of students. Since ADD/ADHD students are never in a majority, their needs are often considered secondary or not considered at all.

Remember the daily assignments you were allotted and had to submit within a set deadline? The stress and frustration that accompanied these assignment completions and the criticism that followed if you were unable to do so were completely de-motivating. Even if you happened to like a subject, there is a high probability that the sheer amount of homework given wore you out. It is like giving an ant a big cube of sugar and expecting it to consume it within the next two minutes.

The ant in my example is symbolic of the fact that ADD/ADHD individuals are often hard workers. You did not complete your homework because it was beyond your capabilities to concentrate for the extended amount of time required to complete it, not because you were too lazy to do so. I am not completely eliminating laziness as a cause! ADD/ADHD individuals can be procrastinators too.

However, not only was the work expected of you beyond your capabilities in school, you were also subject to criticism from teachers, classmates and parents alike. Your self-esteem went for a toss, you were discouraged and frustrated and it wouldn't be surprising if you flew into tantrums at every opportunity.

You were made to sit in one place for hours with classmates who could distract you no end. The teacher probably allotted you a seat near the window and then kept admonishing you for looking out. If you think back to those days, you'll realize that many of your ADD/ADHD symptoms were dealt with in the worst manner ever.

What about now? Now that you are an adult, do you do the same for yourself as others did for you so many years back? You have your life in *your* hands now. You can toss the deflating factors of your environment into the nearest bin and create an inflating atmosphere for yourself. How do you go about doing that?

1. **Escape the assignment trap:** Don't take on more than you can do and have flexible deadlines for its completion, or at least deadlines that will give you sufficient time to complete the task.

2. **Surround yourself with positive people:** Having people who are optimistic and positive about life will give you a similar perspective. Surround yourself with them and avoid negativity or people who are deliberately insulting.

3. **Position yourself:** Where do you sit to work? Ensure that your work table has as few distractions around it as possible. A window or a door close-by will prove to be major distracters; avoid them when you choose your work spot.

4. **Clear that clutter:** ADD/ADHD brains are a collection of a confused mess that is difficult to sort and organize. Being surrounded by clutter in your house or workplace and especially on your worktable will only add to the ADD muddle.

5. **Have a mentor:** Have someone who knows your condition and is willing to help you. Someone you can go to and pour your heart out - someone you can

look to for encouragement - because it is possibly the only thing that ADD/ADHD individuals thrive on.

These are pointers to creating a more inflating environment. You can analyze your specific situation and decide on things you can change or dispose of to ensure a rewarding environment for yourself.

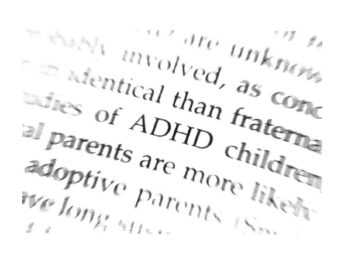

Chapter Thirty One:
When you Spot it, Name it!

"If you have made mistakes, even serious ones, there is always another chance for you. What we call failure is not the falling down but the staying down".

- Mary Pickford

Everyone makes mistakes and those with ADD/ADHD even more so. Why then are we so defensive and refuse to admit our mistakes? A mistake is a mistake, but knowing where it came from can help a lot in preventing a repeat performance.

Those with ADD/ADHD are more prone to bouts of forgetfulness, impulsiveness and hyperactivity. These characteristics can be the root of many of the mistakes you make. Forgetting to deposit a check and eventually ending up losing it is not a small thing. Although you might be tempted to get defensive when asked to account for it, don't! Admit your mistake, instead of spending the next hour trying to defend your actions when there is no excuse at all.

Blaming ADD/ADHD for all your mistakes is a no-no. Firstly, it is just not true that ADD/ADHD is the cause of all the blunders you do. Secondly, by blaming ADD/ADHD for each mistake you make, you start justifying your actions and stop trying to act towards improving them - a trait which is completely undesirable.

Here's what you can do to avoid unnecessary arguments whenever you commit a mistake. First and foremost, recognize that you are at fault. Decide whether it was really your mistake or not. Sometimes, we may be unfairly blamed for something that we didn't do. Try to see clearly who should shoulder the blame. If it was your mistake, try and analyze it to determine where it came from. Was your ADD to blame? If it happened because you were negligent and purposely didn't do something, or landed yourself in a mess you could have stayed away from, don't bring your ADD into the picture.

It helps to have slogans or sayings to go along with your admission. So for instance, if you are at the driver's seat while on your way to a vacation and you end up taking your family on a half-an-hour detour because you were inattentive while at the wheel, you could say *My ADD just made an appearance* or *There goes my ADD again*. Your knee-jerk reaction would be to get frustrated and argue, subconsciously wanting to abort the trip because you did something wrong. Admitting to having done something wrong and a slogan or saying of this sort will help dissipate further argument.

That said, as I mentioned before, a mistake is a mistake and you should not use your ADD to justify all your actions or mis-actions. Forgetting to meet a long-time friend after having promised to do so is not excusable; it was an appointment you made quite some time back. There is a certain amount of responsibility resting on you each time you are given something to do. If you end up blundering and then spend time arguing over your own blunder, you are going to end up irritating and alienating people.

So here's what you do:

1. **Come up with slogans:** Use phrases or sayings like the ones I mentioned above to put your mistakes into perspective. Whenever you do something wrong, recognize where it came from and assign it a short sentence to convey that you've admitted to your mistake.

2. **Inject some humor:** Nothing helps ward off anger and other destructive emotions better than humor. Divert combustible situations to safer grounds by injecting a shot of humor, self-deprecating if need be.

3. **Stop making excuses:** Don't invent excuses for things you did or didn't do. They won't help solve the problem and they surely won't help you.

4. **Avoid unnecessary defensiveness:** Getting defensive at the slightest hint of criticism or reprimand will worsen situations. Let the other person have a chance to convey what they want you to know. Apologize, if it's an apology they need.

5. **Use your "Sorry" with care:** You should say you are sorry for your mistake only if you are sure you won't repeat it again. With your ADD/ADHD in the background, you cannot guarantee that you won't do something you did wrong all over again. Committing the same mistake time and again, and saying sorry each time will indicate that you just don't care and are using the word frivolously.

Its "human" to make mistakes and with ADD/ADHD, even more. So recognize them, admit them, improve them, and move on.

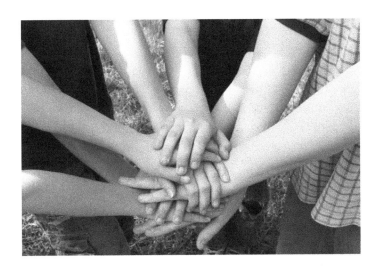

Chapter Thirty Two:
The Secret to Dealing with Other People

"I can find only three kinds of business in the universe: mine, yours, and God's. (For me, the word 'God' means 'reality'. Reality is God, because it rules. Anything that's out of my control, your control, and everyone else's control - I call that God's Business.)"

- Byron Katie.

Most of my adult patients diagnosed with ADD/ADHD have a rich history of conflict with other people. Let's face it, as unique as all human beings are, those with ADD/ADHD behaviors are even more particular, and think quite differently from most.

Naturally, non-ADD/ADHD folks don't always perceive these differences as "creativity", and very often see them as signs of rebellion or downright animosity. When this happens, sparks can fly!

Almost every challenge you will ever experience with another human being will come down to one, or both of the following:

- You are personalizing what they are doing or saying
- You are trying to control them, or resisting being controlled yourself

One of the patterns of communication that dominates here is what I call the "Prisoner/Prison Guard" pattern.

Imagine a movie script that is written from the perspective of a prisoner. The theme is centered on the idea that the prisoner is just trying to serve out his sentence and quietly do his time, however, the prison guards are always making things rough for him. The prisoner is convinced that he is being victimized on a daily basis by the guards - the "bad guys" - who have nothing better to do than make his life miserable.

Now let's imagine reading a different script. This one is written from the perspective of a prison guard.

The main theme this time around is that the poor guards are just trying to make a living; they are risking their lives each day for very low pay, only to be met with the perpetual and incessant onslaught of threats, sarcasm and ridicule by the inmates.

While they might be the ones with the pass-codes and pepper spray, they feel that they are the true victims in this environment, and that the "bad guys" - the prisoners - live to make their lives hell.

What neither of them realize is that the feelings they are experiencing require them to hold onto a particular frame of reference. Neither the prisoner, nor the prison guard can be the victim without thinking of the other as the "bad guy". Likewise, for either of them to feel like a "bad guy", they would have to view the other as the "victim".

Let's take it a step further. If the prison guards were truly convinced of being "victims" of the situation, they would see "bad guys" when they looked at the prisoners, even if the prisoners were model inmates who cooperated and complied with a smile on their faces.

The message I am trying to reinforce here is this: once we have decided to embrace the "victim" position in our lives, we literally have to have "bad guys". I mean, how in the world can you be a "victim" without a "bad guy"?

This means that even when our initial assessment of a person is wrong, and someone we took for being a "bad guy" actually turns out to be a decent human being, if we are still convinced that they have victimized us in some way, we will thrust them into the role of the "bad guy" just to uphold our view of the situation.

And here's the best part, even if someone has treated us somewhat unkindly, if we refuse them the right to perform as the "bad guy", we can simultaneously decline from playing the part of the "victim".

Take some time to consider the far reaching implications of what you have just read. It could change your life or perhaps the life of someone else... The choice is yours, and the ability too.

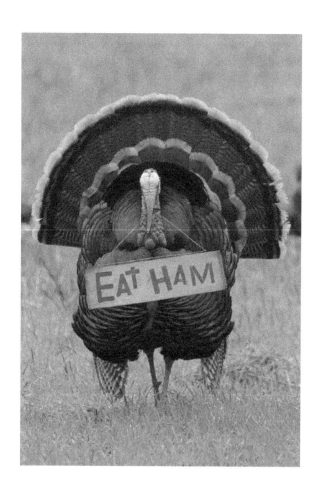

Chapter Thirty Three:
Learn to Make a Great Spaghetti Sauce

"Never do things others can do and will do, if there are things others cannot do or will not do."

- Amelia Earhart.

Spaghetti sauce usually has a tomato base, but before anything else is added, it's simply tomato sauce. It starts to become spaghetti sauce when we start to add *other things*; we start adding onions, sausage, green peppers, or mushrooms.

We start each day with a base of our own, and as we begin to flavor our life with feelings of joy, acceptance, gratitude, or excitement, we begin to flavor the sauce of life.

Just as few people would rave about how delicious a meal of spaghetti and plain tomato sauce would be, we'll find that people who are less than thrilled about their life could usually stand to add some spice to the mix of their daily experience.

As you know, much of what those with ADD/ADHD find irritating is feeling as though they are stuck in one particular, non-productive state of mind and body.

In order for us to really feel like we're living a rich, textured, and meaningful life, we need to be able to access a wide range of emotions, and to be able to vary the intensity of those emotions that we're feeling. And it's these emotions that you can think of as the flavor enhancing ingredients that you add to the spaghetti sauce of your life.

How many different spaghetti sauce recipes can you create, commit to memory, and then whip up from scratch if unexpected guests should happen to drop by for a visit?

When you only have one spaghetti sauce recipe, eating spaghetti could grow tiresome quickly, but when you have lots and lots of recipes, all tasty but distinct, you could feasibly eat plates full of otherwise bland-tasting pasta for weeks on end.

Take a look at the number of emotional and physical states you've limited yourself to experiencing in recent months or years. Then, one at a time, start adding diversity to your day… to your life. See, ADD/ADHD states are a problem, except when they're not.

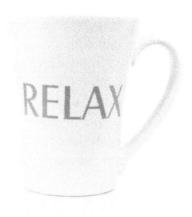

Body and Mind
Looking After Your Physical Health
Means You Will Feel Better

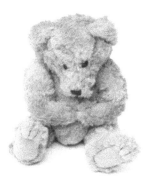

Chapter Thirty Four:
What You're Eating Might Be Eating You

"I saw few die of hunger; of eating, a hundred thousand."

- Benjamin Franklin.

Isn't it funny how the things we do the most - the things we do daily, or several times a day - are often the last things we would think of when attempting to make a connection between a health challenge and its possible cause?

Most people eat 3 meals every day. Some of those meals may be eaten at home, and others might be consumed at a restaurant or a friend's house.

In between meals, there will usually be some kind of snacking going on. This might be in the form of soft drinks, chips, fruit, water, candy bars or any of the other many items available.

So far, I haven't told you anything you didn't already know about the typical eating habits of most people. However, because there is usually so little time between the consumption of one or more food items, and the next time something will be eaten, it can be very difficult to determine what food, or what particular meal, might be causing us to act, think or feel differently.

Adverse reactions can be delayed by a few hours to as much as several days, when we ingest food that has a less than favorable impact. We might, for example, eat something for breakfast that we are allergic to, and yet, it might not start to manifest until after we have eaten lunch. When this occurs, our mind has a tendency to link the feeling we are having with the food item or meal that was most recent.

Is it worth your time to look into possible food allergies? A study at Cornell Medical Center looked at a group of 26 hyperactive kids. After cutting out the most common foods related to food allergens, 19 of these children experienced profound improvements in their hyperactivity.

Because of the potential of a delayed reaction time between the consumption of food and the onset of any symptoms, trying to identify food allergies on your own is often fraught with frustration and lack of progress.

A simple skin-prick test can be a great place to start. A strip with very fine needles and various allergens is pressed against the skin of the back. Anything you are allergic to will cause a small "wheal" or raised area on the skin to appear. This is quick, simple and can trim years off of the process of finding out what foods (or other substances) might be doing you more harm than good.

In some cases, by eliminating the foods you are allergic to, a complete remission of ADD or ADHD symptoms might be experienced. In these cases, the ADD or ADHD diagnosis was likely misdiagnosed, and the true cause of the symptoms was food allergies all along.

Keep in mind, however, that even when the ADD/ADHD diagnosis is accurate, food allergies can play a big role in the frequency and severity of the symptoms.

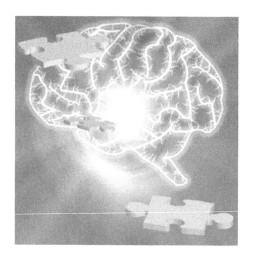

Chapter Thirty Five:
High Protein Diets Proven to Increase Attention and Memory

"Leave your drugs in the chemist's pot if you can heal the patient with food."

- Hippocrates

There are some things that our elders have an uncanny knowledge about. Remember being forced to consume dairy products? How about nuts, eggs, soy and wheat? Do these food groups ring any bells? They are all highly rich in proteins. Science is only now catching up with things we've known for years.

We normally associate high protein consumption with muscular bodies; people going on diets to reduce flab tend to consume food rich in protein. But believe me when

I say that proteins are not "all structure and no function". I have science *and* my own experience to back me on this.

Have you heard of the old adage: "A healthy mind is a healthy body"? Have you ever wished to attain that balance of existence? Proteins are the answer. The fact that proteins help build a strong body is no secret; what is lesser known is that they help improve attention and memory. Is your ADD driving you to lose and misplace things, at times hinting towards a lack of strong memory power? Shift to high protein diets!

Sit back and think about the food you ate today. How much of it was comprised of proteins? The amount of junk food that an average individual consumes is appalling. This food might satiate your taste buds (and maybe your stomach), but all it does is add to the fat reserves in your body. Does your daily diet comprise of a high amount of this "high-fat no-protein" junk? If yes, it's about time you made a conscious effort to incorporate proteins into your diet. Trust me, life will be happier.

Why did I just talk about the relation between proteins and happiness? Let's see. You get up late in the morning, the clock reads 9.00 am and you have to report for work at 10.00. You run to bathroom, take a bath and run out again. Clothes are put on in a hurry, but... wait! Where is the darn watch?! And the socks?! And your tie?! Frustration takes over as you hunt for them. The clock is ticking away... You see what I mean? Proteins lead to increased attention and memory, which lead to organization; organization gives peace... and peace gives happiness.

Since we are on the topic of junk food, there's something I would like to tell you. We know that junk food is bad, irrespective of the fact that we still consume it. But those with ADD and ADHD need to be extra wary of this quick fix. The food additives these products contain have been found to cause an aggravation of ADD symptoms. So the next time you reach for that pack of chips, know that your ADD symptoms are probably going to strike you with full force.

If you want to overcome the discomfort that ADD represents in your life, then you should stop at nothing; and when I say nothing, I don't even mean that there are huge sacrifices you have to make. Wheat, yoghurt, soy, and eggs are products you can easily integrate as a part of your daily diet and take a huge step towards working your way around ADD/ADHD. You can very easily cut down on your junk food consumption. Consuming Omega-3 supplements will not wear you out. These may seem trivial, but you'll appreciate the difference they bring to your life if you actually experience it.

Whoa! Wait just a minute before you run off to stock your kitchen with high protein foods. Remember that this is no quick fix. I know I've mentioned it before, but I'll mention it again; because most ADD patients tend to give up on treatment methods far too quickly (a trait that not only leaves you with your ADD/ADHD intact but also gives rise to a sense of hopelessness - a hopelessness you can do without). Have faith, it's important.

So take it slow and steady. Bringing about a shift in your diet is not a cakewalk; take it one step at a time. It takes at least a month to observe the effects of incorporating high-protein foods in your diet. One month is a short time if you compare it with years of forgetfulness borne of ADD. It is already 9.45 a.m. by the time you fish out your socks. The choice is yours.

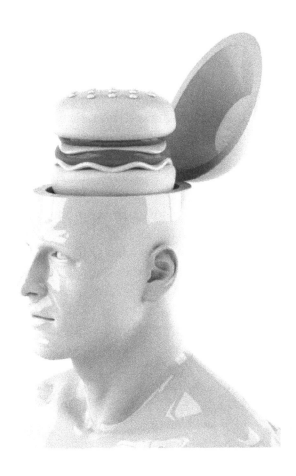

Chapter Thirty Six:
Feeding Your Brain

"The brain is a monstrous, beautiful mess. Its billions
of nerve cells - called neurons - lie in a tangled web that
displays cognitive powers far exceeding any of the silicon
machines we have built to mimic it."

- William F. Allman.

Chances are good that you are not a race car driver. I'm betting that the car you drive is used for the usual stuff; getting back and forth to work, going to the store, dropping loved ones off, etc. Since you don't place extraordinary demands on your car, and don't peg the speedometer on your way to work, the standard spark plugs recommended for your car are ample.

However, the more you desire, in terms of performance, from a car, the more the little things matter. To squeeze a few more horse power from an engine, there are high performance spark plugs that will do just that. It's kind of like this with the human brain.

For many activities, such as passively watching television, the standard American diet is sufficient. Once you have found yourself a contestant on Jeopardy playing for thousands of dollars, writing a thesis, or filing your taxes, though, your brain can benefit from something like a set of high performance spark plugs. Not all activities are equal when it comes to what is required by your brain.

Fortunately, there are several nutritional supplements with a proven track record that will take your very special brain to an even higher level of performance. All of the ones I will be sharing have been extremely effective for many people. My guess would be, however, that not all of them will work for you. They might, but more than likely, you'll find some that really do the trick and some, for whatever reason, just don't do much for you. Know this, expect this, and simply find those that make a difference as quickly as possible; and ditch the ones that don't.

Before I begin talking about specific nutritional supplements in the coming chapters, there's one thing I want to cover. Every now and then someone will ask me, *"how long will I have to take it?"* when they have discovered a supplement that I have suggested is beneficial.

When I inform them that they will only experience the positive effects as long as they are taking the supplement, they sometimes seem upset. *"You mean I'll have to take this everyday to keep my sharper focus?"* "Yes," I reply, *"just as you'll have to breathe and eat everyday to continue to live; it would seem that the things that have the most value are often those that we have to do with frequency."* This usually shifts their thinking to a different - and more healthy - way of looking at things.

So, please understand that these supplements, as profound as the benefits they provide may be, are not a cure, or a one time quick fix. When you experience something you find useful, realize that in order to continue experiencing the clearer thinking, increased energy or other benefit, you'll have to make that supplement a part of your daily routine.

I suspect that you will find that at least one of these nutritional supplements I will be discussing will make a striking difference in how you think and/or feel. Remember, even if the difference is a really BIG difference, it's still best to think in terms of whatever you are doing as being a part - albeit sometimes a very important part - of a much bigger picture.

Let's take a look at the first supplement that may possibly take you to a new level.

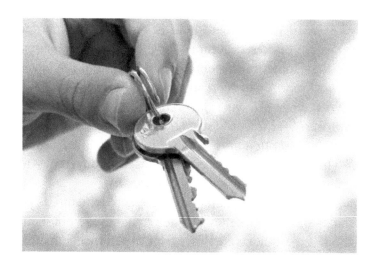

Chapter Thirty Seven:
Omega 3 supplements for
ADD and ADHD

"The wise man should consider that health is the greatest of human blessings. Let food be your medicine."

- Hippocrates.

Since the time they were identified, we've been lead to believe that the cause of ADD and ADHD is not known. And this is used as a justification for the lack of a distinctive cure for these disorders. And over the years you've believed in the same thing and have reconciled yourself to the fact that *"it is hopeless; I am stuck with being hyperactive for the rest of my life"*.

That is far from the truth. Extensive research work carried out on ADD and ADHD indicates that they are not caused exclusively by genetic factors or brain trauma cases. The cause for your ADD condition could be something as simple as an allergy or a deficiency in your diet; speaking of deficiencies, it has been found that most ADD and ADHD patients have low levels of Omega 3 in their diet and consequently, in their body.

Think back to the time you last consumed something rich in Omega-3, like fish or flaxseed oil. How long ago was it? Days... Weeks... or months? Are you consuming enough Omega-3 to eliminate that as a cause for your ADD or ADHD? If not, taking supplements of Omega-3 to combat the disorder could be the way to go.

Omega-3 is a vital fatty acid and is essential for normal growth and development of the brain. Low levels of Omega-3 have been associated with depression, hyperactivity and other symptoms normally associated with attention deficit disorders. I have prescribed Omega-3 supplements to many of my patients with remarkable results. Nearly 80 percent observed a positive effect within four weeks.

Note: I said *four* weeks. Patience is a virtue; you've waited months (even years) for a cure; don't go looking for a quick fix remedy for the disorder. You might observe a positive effect within a couple of weeks following initiation of Omega-3 consumption, but remember that the supplements have to be taken continuously, unless you incorporate Omega-3 into your daily diet.

It started with our parents. Then magazines, radio, television, and even Internet, harping on every chance they get, about consuming a "balanced diet," until we finally decided "enough is enough". We had the balanced diet components studied down to the very last letter. The question here is, how much of it did we implement? The effect a balanced diet can have, by virtue of being either present or absent in our lifestyle, is tremendous. Take Omega-3 as a prime example. A major chunk of ADD/ADHD cases would be non-existent if the food people consumed was properly balanced and contained all the essential elements required by our body.

You've heard about the old lady who can't find her spectacles. She searches all over the house for them, turning over drawers, bed sheets and shelves. She even checks the fridge and the shoe racks. Imagine her distress; the poor lady did so like to read! No points for guessing where her glasses were; they were on top of her head the whole time and she forgotten about them!

Although this tale is often used to explain the search for God, or conscience, or how one need not look far and wide to find what they are looking for, I feel it is a tale for all situations where the solution to our problems lies right under our noses. What I want to emphasize here is that the solution to so many of our problems is so close at hand, yet we tend to overlook it all the time, wandering farther and farther away in our quest for the perfect answer.

You go from one doctor to another, and then make an appointment with a psychologist, then move on to join a mental exercise class, all the while looking for the elusive cure for your ADD or ADHD. How about walking over to the medical store across the street and buying a couple of Omega-3 supplement containers? Your attention deficit disorder could well be a simple case of Omega-3 deficit.

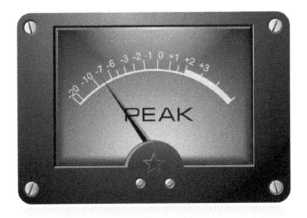

Chapter Thirty Eight:
Tyrosine for a Mental Pick-Me-Up

"To enjoy good health, to bring true happiness to one's family, to bring peace to all, one must first discipline and control one's own mind. If a man can control his mind he can find the way to Enlightenment, and all wisdom and virtue will naturally come to him."

- Buddha.

Have you heard of those molecules in your body called neurotransmitters? These small molecules serve in the conduction of nerve impulses between the different neurons of the brain and those distributed in the spinal cord. Why am I telling you this?

Imagine a nation which has no modern means of communication and is dependent on messengers to deliver information within and outside its boundaries. These messengers have to be specially trained to deliver their messages to the proper recipient in the shortest span of time. What would happen if there weren't enough messengers? Everything would be delivered at a sluggish pace and this would eventually affect the functioning of the entire nation.

Now, substitute brain and neurotransmitters for nation and messengers respectively. Get what I mean? In most individuals with ADD/ADHD, neurotransmitters are in extreme short supply, which explains the inattentiveness and depression. But fret not; shortage of neurotransmitters is not equivalent to life-long ADD. In fact, if this is the only cause for your ADD/ADHD, you have practically nothing to worry about; it is when there are numerous causes that some complications can arise.

These neurotransmitters are made of amino acids, like glutamine, glycine and tyrosine, the subunits of proteins. Consuming high-protein food can help in the production of neurotransmitters, thus helping the brain tide over their shortage. If you've read articles on natural methods to overcome ADD/ADHD, you will have noticed that the amino acid Tyrosine makes a regular appearance. What sets it apart?

Have you ever had stressful situations in your life? Sorry, wrong question; everyone's had stressful situations in their lives. What I want to know is what is your reaction to the stress? Did you fight the stress or slip into depression due to your inability to cope? If you did the latter (don't worry, you're not alone), tyrosine can help you. Here's how.

Tyrosine is a precursor for three neurotransmitters; dopamine, norepinephrine and serotonin. Dopamine and norepinephrine regulate motor functions and hormone release. In addition, dopamine is also responsible for regulating emotions. Your perception of well-beingstems from the release of the neurotransmitter serotonin.

Since dopamine and norepinephrine are involved in the regulation of motor functions, their deficiency leads to fatigue and muscular weakness, as reported by many ADD/ADHD patients.

Those who are depressed feel they are no good, their self esteem and emotional health takes a downward dip. There's nothing like a good dose of serotonin to restore your sense of well-being and bring good cheer.

I am sure you've heard of the hormone adrenaline, often used in common parlance to denote the response or need for thrill (*"The rollercoaster ride gave me an adrenaline high!"*). Adrenaline is the hormone released in response to perceived or real stress. Tyrosine helps build up the stock of adrenaline in your body.

The beneficial effects of Tyrosine are not restricted to fighting stress alone, although that is no mean feat by itself. Think of any symptom associated with ADD/ADHD and there is a high probability that tyrosine would be able to alleviate it. Lack of discipline? Tyrosine is the answer. Mood instability? Tyrosine again. Inattentiveness? Increase your tyrosine consumption. Memory loss? Look no further than tyrosine. So important and effective is this amino acid in the treatment of ADD/ADHD that I had no qualms about dedicating a whole chapter for it, after having already covered high-protein diets.

Dairy products, fish, meat and beans are all good sources of tyrosine. You could alternatively opt for tyrosine supplements. I'd recommend a dosage of 1,000-1,500 mg to overcome ADD/ADHD symptoms. Also, ensure that you take multi-vitamin supplements along with tyrosine, to enable its conversion to brain chemicals.

What are neurotransmitters? Can't remember? Tyrosine is the way to go. Life is good, but with ADD, stress, fatigue and all, why not make it better?

Healthy FOCUS

Chapter Thirty Nine:
What the French Know about Mental Clarity: Pycnogenol

"Our mental and emotional diets determine our overall energy levels, health, and well-being to a far greater extent than most people realize. Every thought and feeling, no matter how big or small, impacts our inner energy reserves."

- Doc Childre and Howard Martin,

The HeartMath Solution.

If you have ADD or ADHD, there is a good chance that mental clarity is not one of your strong points. Those with ADD are sharp and intelligent, but when it comes to clarity of thoughts and organization of, as they put it, the mess in their brain, they have nothing to boast about. Think Thomas Elva Edison, Albert Einstein or Mozart - intelligent and creative yet so distracted; constantly jumping from one train of thought to another. You begin to see the lack of mental clarity hidden behind the genius. All of them probably had ADD/ADHD.

Why do you think those with ADD/ADHD lack clarity of thoughts? Think of a transparent glass filled with crystal clear water. Now if I were to add some amount of soil to it, what would happen to its clarity? A similar sort of explanation can be given for mental confusion and disorganization. The brain is an awesome organ which works better than the best machine on earth. When toxins invade it, or are produced due to certain reactions, it cannot maintain its perfect functioning.

You must have heard of radicals in conjunction with cancer and aging. However, their effect is not restricted only to cancerous cells or wrinkled skin, these radicals can affect practically every cell in your body and the brain (which is protected from most damaging forces by the blood-brain barrier) is also vulnerable to radicals.

There are also certain compounds in the body, either ingested and retained, or produced due to certain metabolic reactions that are harmless to other cells of the body yet can cause damage to cells of the brain if they succeed in crossing the blood-brain barrier.

It's time to dissolve some alum in the water - we want the clarity back! So, what can be done to enhance mental clarity if you have ADD/ADHD?

Pycnogenol, a complex of several compounds obtained from the bark of the French maritime bark or grape seeds, is an extremely strong antioxidant. Know what that means? I bet you do; it can be the alum in your body, neutralizing the radicals, preventing further damage. If radicals can cross the blood brain barrier, so can Pycnogenol.

It helps get rid of the radicals in your brain and suddenly the world is so much clearer. As one patient put it, *"it's like putting on a new pair of spectacles"*. Not only can Pycnogenol fight radicals, it can also detoxify your brain of those compounds I just mentioned.

Besides detoxification, Pycnogenol protects your blood vessels and increases circulation. Now you may ask, *"How does this have anything to do with mental clarity?"* You sure are in need of some clarity! Increased circulation means increased blood flow, increased blood flow means more blood flowing to and from the brain. More blood to the brain means more nutrients, which translates into more energy and better thought processes. More blood from the brain leads to faster disposal of waste produced in the brain… Talk about efficient clean ups!

The clearer your brain, the better your concentration and organization. No more mess in the brain! Unlike most other supplements which take quite some time to work, Pycnogenol is very rapid in action. Research has shown that on consumption, Pycnogenol is rapidly absorbed and functions as an extremely strong cell detoxifier.

Recent studies further demonstrate that Pycnogenol may also have an excitatory effect on the "feel good" neurotransmitters; dopamine and norepinephrine. It can thus help those with ADD/ADHD combat stress which they are otherwise very vulnerable to. Various nutrients that have been proven to help ADHD treatment, such as selenium, copper and zinc, are delivered to the brain via Pycnogenol.

Many ADD/ADHD patients who have taken Pycnogenol have reported an increase in productivity stemming from a newly acquired ability to focus. A dosage of 1mg/pound a day should offer all these benefits.

Pycnogenol has proven its case and I've passed my verdict - have you? A clearer mind and a clearer world is within your reach… Reach out; your brain will thank you.

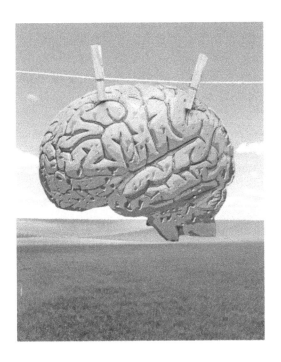

Chapter Forty:
Better "Thinko" with Gingko

"We are coming to understand health not as the absence of disease, but rather as the process by which individuals maintain their sense of coherence (i.e. sense that life is comprehensible, manageable, and meaningful) and ability to function in the face of changes in themselves and their relationships with their environment."

- Aaron Antonovsky.

Have you heard of the Gingko Biloba? It is one of the oldest species on earth. I can hear you saying, "What is something so ancient doing in a book on ADD/ADHD?"

Being ancient has its benefits. It gives people a lot of time to do research on you, and the Gingko Biloba has been researched in extreme detail. So, what are its benefits, from an ADD/ADHD perspective?

1. **Increased cerebral blood flow**: The brain makes up a small part of your body, yet consumes the largest amount of energy. It is therefore in need of constant nutrient replenishment and waste removal. If you observe sluggish behavior in an individual, as is noted in some ADD/ADHD cases, you can be sure that the individual has a sluggish blood circulation. You see, the slower the blood moves, the lesser the amount of nutrients available to the brain in a certain span of time. And the brain can work at its fastest only when its nutrient and energy demands are met.

2. **Irritable no more**: Gingko can help people with ADD/ADHD fight irritability and frustration. The irritable nature of ADD/ADHD patients is quite understandable, but you need not let it get the better of you. Having to sort through the disorganization of your brain can be challenging job; therefore having a multi-spectrum treatment method can help enormously. Gingko in conjunction with Pycnogenol can tremendously help to overcome irritable behavior.

3. **Inattention be gone**: That ADD/ADHD patients have trouble retaining information is common knowledge. Concentrating on tasks is no picnic for most with ADD. Gingko helps overcome this inability.

4. **The "Smart Drug"**: Those with ADD/ADHD are recognized as highly intelligent and creative, but how will that intelligence come to the surface if you are not focused and can't shape a productive result out of all your intelligent and creative thoughts? That is where Ginkgo comes into the picture, by

helping you put your intelligence down on paper. Ginkgo helps make your *"Eureka!"* moments a frequent occurrence.

5. **Defy the defiant brain**: ADD/ADHD encourages defiance, which can be very tiresome to those you interact with and even to yourself. It is not impossible to fight your defiant side, but it sure is difficult. Gingko helps overcome defiant behavior and makes life more peaceful.

The amount prescribed on the bottles tends to be too low to show any considerable effect. I'd recommend a dosage of 60-120 mg twice a day. I will take this as my cue to repeat my mantra: Patience is the key. Give up too soon and you'd be better off not having started this mode of treatment. It is an herbal medicine, perfected by nature over the years; you cannot expect it to work on you within a span of a few hours. It may not be quickest cure on earth, but it is considerably better than the quick-fix, side-effect-giving, short-term, over-the-counter medicines. It has a permanent result *and* is without side effects, if taken within the dosage recommended.

Being able to survive on earth for billions of years is no mean feat, especially when all other species around you are getting extinct and God is playing mischief sending earthquake after earthquake, volcano eruption after eruption, and hurricane after hurricane. What was needed for survival then, wasfaith, belief and determination. Gingko Biloba did it and has, to the present millennia, embodied all the qualities needed for a meaningful survival. It can pass them on to you. It asks for only three things: faith, belief and determination.

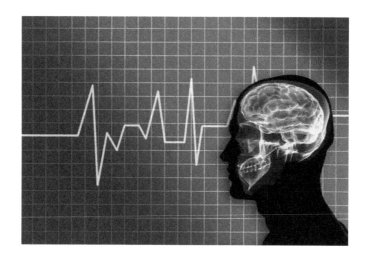

Chapter Forty One:
More Energy, Sharper Focus and Less Pain...What More Could You Want?

"Anguish of mind has driven thousands to suicide; anguish of body, none. This proves that the health of the mind is of far more consequence to our happiness than the health of the body, although both are deserving of much more attention than either of them receive."

- Charles Caleb Colton.

Every one of us has a Dr. Jekyll and a Mr. Hyde side to us. Nothing and nobody is 100 percent good or useful; neither will you find anything or anybody 100 percent bad or useless. Are you wondering what I mean by "nothing" and how a "thing" can have two sides? I mean if a thing is useful, it is useful and if it is harmful, it's harmful, right? Wrong! To give you an example: how many times have you heard, read and spread the fact that water is good and one should have 10-12 glasses of water a day? But is this really true? There are some for whom this amount is high enough to cause electrolyte imbalance in their body.

In this chapter, I'll introduce you to a molecule which has no apparent Mr. Hyde face, rather it has three Dr. Jekyll sides. Curious? Here we go.

If chemistry is your forte, you might be aware that some compounds have two different chemical forms, D and L, which can exist in combination with each other or individually. Often, only one of the two forms is active and if both can act chemically it is very rare that both will produce useful results. Consider the hormone Thyroxine, it exists in the D and L form, of which only the L form is active and the D form is inactive. In cases of Thyroxine deficiencies, administering the D form will not have any effect; you will have to inject the L form.

The molecule I am going to introduce you to is Phenylalanine, an amino acid. It exists in the D and L forms and is of the rare type I mentioned above; i.e. both its D and L forms are useful and active. In fact D, L and DL Phenylalanine, all three serve important functions in our body; functions that should be of special interest to those with ADD/ADHD.

Does the word "endorphin" ring a bell? Think chocolate and you'll know what I am talking about. Endorphins are opiates that our body naturally produces. Know the feeling you get after eating dark chocolate, that "feel-good" and "high" factor is due to the increase in endorphins flowing in your body. D-Phenylalanine helps maintain constant blood levels of endorphins and thus help you tide over pain.

Moreover, D-Phenylalanine is responsible for maintaining blood levels of compounds called enkephalins. Before you go *"enkepha...what?"*, these compounds increase mental alertness, akin to caffeine. The more alert you are, the sharper your focus on the task at hand will be and better will be your results.

Let's look at its second Dr. Jekyll face. The L-form is also involved in increasing mental alertness. It regulates your mood and therefore those of you who slip into depression at the slightest sight of stress, can benefit immensely from its consumption. How does it work? I've already covered tyrosine in the previous chapter; L-phenylalanine is the precursor of tyrosine, and an indirect precursor of dopamine and norepinephrine. So now you know where the anti-depressant properties come from.

The DL form for most compounds is an inactive state of existence; however DL-Phenylalanine exhibits the effects of both D and L forms of Phenylalanine, thus acting as pain-reliever, energy booster and mental stimulator all thrown into one.

What makes Phenylalanine so potent is its ability to cross the blood-brain barrier and cause a direct effect on the brain cells. Natural sources of Phenylalanine include milk, fish, meat, cheese and soybeans. You can opt for Phenylalanine supplements if you wish to. I'd recommend a dose of 400mg three times each day on an empty stomach. Again, here comes the reminder: patience is the key. It will take at least one to two weeks for the effects to become apparent, so wait and watch, don't start and stop.

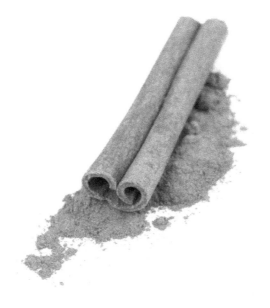

Chapter Forty Two:
Cinnamon for Life?

"If I'd known I was going to live so long, I'd have taken better care of myself."

- Leon Eldred.

There is a fair amount of research indicating that blood glucose challenges and ADD/ADHD often go hand in hand. Not only can this wreak havoc on energy levels, but it can also play a big part in unwanted weight gain, and/or difficulty losing weight.

I came to discover the importance of keeping stable blood sugar levels for cardiovascular health in an interesting way. Little did I know it would also result in an almost effortless weight loss of 15 pounds over the next 4 months.

I was aware that there was some heart disease on both sides of the family with one side, in particular having a fair amount of diabetes. So, I began looking through the research available on using supplements to stabilize and lower blood sugar levels. What I found interested me, but what I experienced was nothing short of amazing.

(You do not have to have diabetes or a history of diabetes in your family to benefit from this. Most people become somewhat insulin resistant as they age, and anything that increases your insulin sensitivity, will not only contribute to you cardiovascular health, but make losing weight and maintaining it MUCH easier).

I began taking cinnamon capsules with every meal. I have not eaten a single meal, in over a year, without also taking my cinnamon/chromium capsules. (I take Walgreen's Cinnamon with Chromium - Chromium is a mineral that also assists in metabolizing sugar).

Cost is not a significant factor; cinnamon is a relatively inexpensive supplement. I plan to take it with every meal for the rest of my life, just as I have something to drink with every meal, and will for the rest of my life. Not a big deal, and very, very simple and easy to do.

The result? My fasting blood glucose is lower. I no longer get sleepy or tired after eating a meal that is heavier in carbohydrates than usual. I lost about 15 pounds - most of it the stubborn stuff around my waist that had never been responsive to anything else. (With insulin resistance, the waist and hips tend to harbor fat that is more resistant than other areas of the body).

Is cinnamon the "magic bullet"? No, it's not. However, for some people, it can truly make a big enough difference to make it an essential part of the overall simple and easy plan.

I've witnessed the impact of stabilizing blood sugar/ glucose levels on learning, thinking, and simply functioning in everyday life, and, I must say, it's quite impressive.

By the way, you might find it interesting to know how this discovery was made. Like so many cool things that come to be, the effectiveness of cinnamon on blood glucose was discovered by accident.

Scientists at the USDA's Human Nutrition Research Center in Maryland were exploring various foods, noting the impact they had on blood glucose levels after being eaten.

While testing apple pie - a food they expected to wreak havoc on blood glucose levels - they discovered that the blood glucose levels of those who had eaten this delicious desert... actually IMPROVED!

Later studies showed that 6 grams of cinnamon a day lowered the pre-cinnamon blood glucose average of 234 mg/ dl to 166 mg/dl, triglycerides decreased up to 30%, and LDL cholesterol dropped by as much as 27%.

Now, make sure we are clear about something... I'm NOT telling you to run out and eat apple pie right now... walk ... I don't want you to fall on your way to the kitchen. Liberal shakes of cinnamon, please ;)

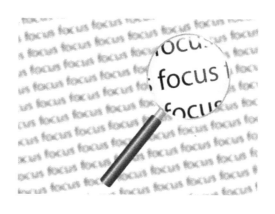

Chapter Forty Three:
The "Fly to Japan" Strategy

"Man's troubles are rooted in extreme attention to senses, thoughts, and imagination. Attention should be focused internally to experience a quiet body and a calm mind."

- Buddha.

I'll never forget the conversation I had with a friend who had lived in Guam for a couple of years. He said *"You know, after the first flight from Portland, Oregon to Tokyo, en route to Guam, I was amazed at how much focused work I was able to get done in the 16 hours between Portland and Narita Airport, in Tokyo."*

He continued, *"At first, I thought it was a coincidence, assuming that it was simply the result of having nothing else to do during the flight. But then, on a return flight to the States, this time taking the Hawaii path home, I was far from being as centered as I had been on the Tokyo flight.*

One week later, on my way back to Guam, and going through Tokyo once again, that same 'Zen' like state returned. About 30 minutes before we landed in Tokyo, I had a 'Eureka' moment; it dawned on me that because the flights routed through Tokyo served a very authentic and distinctly different green tea, I opted for this instead of my usual infusion of a continual flow of coffee.

Just moments before I had been flipping through a fitness magazine and happened upon a blurb about something called L-Theanine; a substance found in green tea that can produce profound states of relaxation without causing drowsiness. The rest is history. And I've been using this accidental discovery for creating laser-like focus for several years now."

My friend had discovered the focus enhancing properties that millions of green tea drinkers from around the world have experienced for centuries.

Placebo effect? Hardly; a study that was published in the Brain Topography Journal concluded that L-Theanine exhibited a measurable effect on the brainwaves of participants taking 250 mg of the supplement each day. Most notably, an increase in alpha-wave activity, resulting in a significant increase in mental focus. Several other studies have detected the increase in alpha-wave activity as well.

Alpha-waves equal a quiet mind, and a quiet mind is a mind that finds it easier to focus and is less likely to experience the intrusion of distracting thoughts. In short, anything we can do to create more alpha brainwaves is going to give us a "clearer" head and allow us to zero in on a task with far more concentration and energy. Consuming L-Theanine will do just that - and fast - the effect is felt within 30 minutes.

Should you take an L-Theanine supplement or simply drink green tea? Considering that most green tea sold in the United States contains about 10 mg per cup, you'd have to drink 10 - 20 cups to get what scientists consider a therapeutic dose of L-Theanine. The higher grade teas, like the one my friend was drinking on his flight to Tokyo contain as much as 50 mg per cup, so 2 - 4 cups of this stuff was enough to pop his brain into focus mode.

If drinking tea isn't your thing, many good L-Theanine supplements are available in 50 - 200 mg capsules so you can light up your "thinker" without firing up the tea pot.

Remember, it's not the "Holy Grail" we are looking for; the idea is to find several things you can do that make a difference, and then to do them all. Find the things that work, use the things that work, and repeat daily!

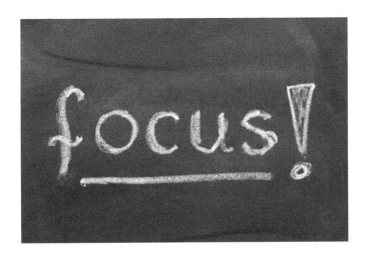

Chapter Forty Four:
Sniffing Your Way to a Clearer
Mind and Sharper Focus

"Those herbs which perfume the air most delightfully, not passed by as the rest, but, being trodden upon and crushed, are three; that is, burnet, wild thyme and watermints. Therefore, you are to set whole alleys of them, to have the pleasure when you walk or tread."

- Francis Bacon.

If you haven't heard the term "aromatherapy" you have probably been living in a cave for the last 25 years. Every isle of the grocery store has at least one product that somehow incorporates the use of scent in its marketing plan. Your olfactory senses (sense of smell) are wired directly to the emotional seat of your brain - the limbic system. This is one reason why aromatherapy can be so helpful.

There is one particular scent that I will discuss; one that you may have never even heard of: Vetiver.

Dr. Terry Friedman found that aromatherapy could be amazingly effective if the right scent or essential oil was used. Curious about what he might be able to do for wondering minds, he had kids sniffing various scents over a two year period. There were 40 children in this study; 20 with ADD/ADHD who did not sniff the essential oil scents, and 20 kids with ADD/ADHD who did.

Once a month, Dr. Friedman would re-access to see how they were doing. What he found was staggering.

The Lavender oil was helpful; performance was about 50% better when they sniffed this scent each time they felt they their mind was wondering. Cedarwood shot their performance up just over 80%. Vetiver, however, blasted performance scores by a whopping 100%.

The most interesting aspect of the study was what was observed happening with their brainwaves. When they inhaled the Vetiver scent, their brainwaves returned to a calm and centered wave pattern.

Am I suggesting that Vetiver oil is a cure all and that you should drop everything else and just sniff this oil every day? No. You will remember though, that I did suggest very early on, that you should incorporate anything that holds promise, keeping what works and ditching the things that don't.

Since most essential oil bottles are about the size of a tube of lip gloss or chap-stick, it should certainly be easy enough to carry this nostril flaring brain soother (Vetiver oil) in your pocket and pull it out a few times a day to inhale deeply. Another nice thing is the cost; a bottle of Vetiver essential oil can be purchased for $8 - $20 and should last a long time.

Don't take Dr. Friedman's word for it, for less than the price of a ticket to a movie, you can do what I always suggest - find out for yourself.

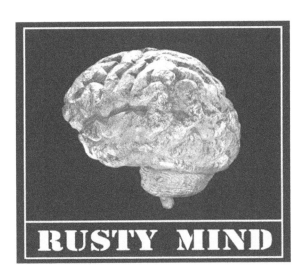

RUSTY MIND

Chapter Forty Five:
Cleaning Up Your Brain with
N-Acetyl-Cysteine (NAC)

"If a man does not keep pace with his companions, perhaps it is because he hears a different drummer. Let him step to the music which he hears, however measured or far away."

- Henry David Thoreau

By now, it should come as no surprise, that as human beings, we are all about rewards. Problem is, we can link some pretty crazy behaviors up with the idea, concept and feeling of "reward". Compulsive gamblers, for example, have gambling hooked into the reward circuitry of their brain; they hit the casino, and sit down to a game of black jack, and BAM….the pleasure center of the brain fires off.

If you or a loved one are dealing with ADHD, there is almost certainly a very similar behavior/reward circuitry connection going on.

In a recent study, people who were struggling with the life wrecking impact of compulsive gambling were given NAC-N-Acetyl- Cysteine, and amino acid that plays a role in a chemical in the human brain connected with the reward circuitry-glutamate. The results were staggering.

Of all of the compulsive gamblers in the study, 60 %, or 6 of every 10 people, experienced a marked reduction in their cravings for hitting the casino, when taking NAC. But here is where it really gets interesting. Those who did well with NAC in this study, went on to participate in a second study; half continued to get NAC, the other half got the famed placebo, or "sugar" pill.

In this follow on study, 83% of those taking NAC continued with the benefits of reduced gambling urges, but 72% of those getting the placebo, were back to gambling like wild, once again.

Why is NAC so effective at controlling urges and compulsive cravings? It's likely because of NAC's incredible and specific antioxidant capabilities.

Below are some of the other remarkable issues NAC has been used to effectively address:

* To break up mucus and prevent recurrence of chronic bronchitis
* Used in hospital emergency settings-at very high levels-to treat acetaminophen poisoning
* To protect the kidneys from iopromide-contrast "dye"-commonly used in conjunction with CT scans
* To reduce the production of cells associated with colon polyps, and possibly diminish the risk of colon cancer
* Preventing kidney damage that can occur when undergoing coronary angiography, as a result of contrast

"dye" utilized to better view coronary arteries. (One study showed an 86% reduction of kidney damage)

So, what do these things have to do with ADD or ADHD? Quite a bit, actually; both ADD and ADHD are often associated with things like chemical sensitivities, allergens, and things like mercury toxicity etc. With its proven ability to detoxify and protect, NAC is one supplement that might very well be worth implementing.

Now, as if the anti-oxidant aspect of NAC wasn't enough, a recent German study found that NAC has another HUGE benefit. This study, published in the Journal of Molecular Medicine, states that when participants were dosed at 600 mg per day-with NAC-for a period of 8 weeks, they lost 5% of their total body fat. The researchers theorize that this result comes from NAC's ability by decreasing insulin's ability to interface with fat cells.

Because spikes in blood sugar, or low blood sugar can mimic, or exacerbate the symptoms of ADD and ADHD, clearly, anything that helps stabilize glucose metabolism is going to be a friend to most anyone with either of these challenges. At the very least, it can support your cardiovascular health.

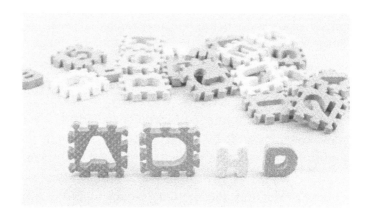

Chapter Forty Six:
Crossing Over

"There is no scientific study more vital to man than the
study of his own brain. Our entire view of the
universe depends on it."

- Francis H.C. Crick.

In the last decade the term "whole brain learning"
has become more and more common. In short, whole brain
learning means that various methods are used to engage
more of both hemispheres of the brain for enhanced learning.

Countless light and sound machines and other so-
phisticated devices exist for the purpose of helping you to
quickly activate more of your brain on each side. However,
I'm going to share a method you can use to do the same
thing for free.

When someone has a stroke that injures and destroys
tissue in the right side of their brain, it's the left side of

their body that is affected. If the stroke is on the left side, the right side of their body will take the brunt of the injury.

We all know how exercise can ignite your brain, flooding it with more oxygen and dopamine, but you don't necessarily need to join the gym to give yourself an extra boost. One simple change is all that is required.

By doing what are called "cross-lateral" movements, you can call more of the gray glob between your ears into action. A cross-lateral movement is any movement that involves crossing any arm or leg across your mid-line, or the center of your body.

Imagine a line that starts between your eyes and runs right down the center of your body, all the way to the floor.

When you are out for a walk, for example, simply swing your arms in a slightly exaggerated manner so that they swing over and across this imaginary line. When your right arm crosses, it activates your left hemisphere; when your left arm crosses, the right hemisphere lights up.

Okay, maybe you've been in class all day, or doing something at the office and haven't had the opportunity to go for your daily walk or run. Would you still like to bring more of your brain into the game? What do you do?

In 60 seconds you can fire up your brain without ever leaving your seat. Place your right hand on your right thigh and your left hand on the left thigh. Now, in a slow rhythmic motion, lightly grab your nose with your right hand, while simultaneously grabbing your right ear with your left hand. Now switch; grab your nose with your left hand and your left ear with your right hand.

At first it will be a little awkward and clumsy, but after just a few times, you'll get a feel for it and be able to increase your speed. Speed, however, is not the goal; the goal is to simply do a minute or two of repeated cross-lateral movements.

Again, because this seems so simple (and it is) some people will initially think *"what can that possibly do?"* My answer? More than you can imagine! I've seen cross-lateral movements - when used daily - change people's lives significantly. Give yourself at least a week of a minimum of 5 minutes of cross-lateral movements each day, and then decide for yourself.

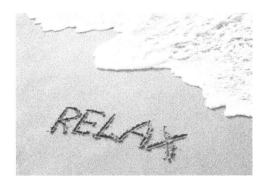

Chapter Forty Seven:
The Relaxation Paradox

"Man is so made that he can only find relaxation from
one kind of labor by taking up another."

- Anatole France.

I cringe every time I hear someone in the field of education suggesting that students should learn to relax deeply in order to enhance their ability to learn and remember.

While it's true that states of fear, frustration and confusion can undercut your best effort to take in new material and have access to it later, deep relaxation is not the answer.

To be at your best and prime your brain for new and improved levels of learning, the following states are the most useful:

- Curiosity
- Excitement
- Anticipation

While there may be an element of relaxation within each of these states, I think you'll agree that you wouldn't associate curiosity, excitement or anticipation with deep relaxation.

I'm going share something with you that will allow you to shift into these states more easily, but first, let me ask you a question: did you know that what position your body is in (body language) makes a huge difference to the state you are in and, therefore, your ability to learn effectively?

I just revealed one of the keys for accessing the learning state. When I said I was going to ask you a question, it put your brain into a higher "alert" status.

When we know we are going to be asked a question, we want to be sure to get all of the information and process the question accurately so we'll be more likely to answer it correctly.

While your brain was in that slightly more attentive state, I delivered a key idea: that the way you use your body and the position that it's in plays a huge role in your ability to learn more effectively. (And I just used another method while explaining the last one - repetition - more on this one in another chapter).

By repeating the statement "body language and the position of your body play a huge role in your ability to learn more effectively" while explaining the previous mind shifting method, I got to share the information a second time. Ooops, I guess I used it this time too; that makes three!

Want to know the body language secret for instantly accessing an ultra-powerful learning state? Here it is: (Read this and then DO it).

1. Lean forward
2. Open your eyes wider
3. Slightly nod your head "yes"
4. Tilt your head to one side just a bit

If you do all of these things at once and don't notice a difference, you might want to call 911! Your body and mind are part of the same unit; there is no "mind body connection"; they are ONE. Change your body radically and you change your mental and emotional states radically.

If you want to retain more of what someone is telling you, or of an email you are reading, or virtually anything else, put your body in the position it would be in if you were in a massive state of anticipation; as if you had already matched the first five numbers of the Powerball lottery and were waiting to hear the final number.

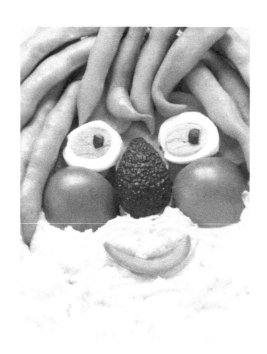

Chapter Forty Eight:
How Does Your Garden Grow?

Many parents around the world have become more and more aware of the growing problem of childhood obesity and juvenile diabetes. In an attempt to guide their children towards a brighter future-one with fewer chronic health problems-some parents are pushing more fruits and vegetables at meal time. Interestingly, this may be causing more problems, for some, than solutions.

A recent study at found that pesticides found in minute amounts in many fruits and vegetables are being found in many children across the United States. These children are twice as likely to be diagnosed with ADHD.

1,139 children were participants in this study. Their urine was collected and analyzed; byproducts from many pesticides, also called *organophospahtes* were measured. Similar studies had been done in the past, and the relationship between high levels of pesticides and impaired cognitive functioning was known. However, studies done in the past had targeted high risk groups, like those working on farms, and others who came into close contact with pesticides. This study, though, looked at a more general sample of the population.

Why are pesticides such a problem when they wind up in our body? It's simple; by design, pesticides are created to target and damage the nervous system of insects and pests. Unfortunately, they also damage the human nervous system. *"That's how they kill pests."* says a researcher at the University of Montreal, Maryse Bouchard, Ph.D. According to Bouchard, pesticides work on certain brain chemicals that are intimately linked to those implicated in ADHD.

Shockingly, measurable levels of pesticides were found in up to 28% of fruits and vegetables, according to the U.S. Department of Agriculture. So, what are we to do, if we wish to avoid taking in "insect killer" when trying to take care of our health?

Bouchard suggests getting your vegetables from places like your local farmers market, or buying organic. Studies have found that even if the vegetables you buy at a farmers market are not organic, they tend to contain far less pesticides.

Here's another idea; what if you were to grow some vegetables of your own? Even if you have a very limited space, there are many vegetables that can be grown with relative ease in a very small area. I can tell you from experience that the taste is so much better, and the fact that you can eat a vegetable that you are 100% certain is "clean" is a very comforting feeling as well.

While the phrase "you are what you eat" may be a stretch, it would be fair to say "you'll be influenced, for better, or worse, by what you eat"

Start to investigate your options for getting fruits and vegetables that are as close to pesticide free as possible. Do you have a friend or neighbor with enough space on their property that might be interested in a garden co-op, where you do the work, and share your harvest with them? The possibilities are many, and the flavors, delicious!

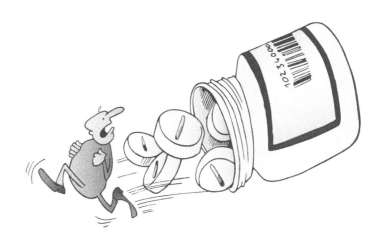

Chapter Forty Nine:
A New Look at an Old Topic

"The best non-pharmacological treatment for ADD
is exercise, sex, and humor."

- Dr. Ned Hallowell,
Co-author of Driven to Distraction.

For years now, we've been inundated with one study after another about how important exercise is for staving off heart disease. Suddenly, however, new research is emerging each day on the power of exercise for improving cognitive function and delaying dementia and Alzheimer's disease.

The problem with exercise and heart disease is that many people don't *feel* a big difference. The protective aspects are there, but because they don't feel a huge and *immediate* payoff, it can begin to feel like a waste of time.

Yes, they know that walking or running each day is silently doing wonderful things for their health - or hope that it is - but most people are far more motivated by getting the rewards NOW.

Thankfully, ADD/ADHD is something that responds rather quickly to exercise. Those taking part in a study that examined the impact of exercise on decision making improved their decisiveness by 11% over the 3 month study by walking for 45 minutes, 3 times per week.

Professor Arthur F. Kramer, a scientist at the Beckman Institute for Advanced Science and Technology, found a number of benefits for the brain that resulted from aerobic exercise.

When you walk, run, play tennis, hike, or do anything else that gets your heart rate up for a sustained period of time, increased levels of oxygen and dopamine race to your brain, increasing focus and bringing a sense of clarity and heightened attention.

Interesting, when our thinking is at its "fuzziest" we tend to conclude that what we need is more rest. While rest is important, far more people suffer from too little exercise than from too much. If you don't exercise at the current time, when you find your mind a little cloudy, go for a brisk walk.

When you're through, re-evaluate your mental status. Chances are good - very good - that you'll find your thinking has become much sharper and that your ability to focus has increased significantly.

Once you've noticed the link between exercise and razor sharp thinking, you'll find it much easier to get into the habit of exercising 3 - 4 days a week.

The benefits of exercise are numerous, but you already knew that. I'm not going to tell you all about how exercise will help your heart, reduce your risk of stroke and various cancers, or how it can supercharge your sex life; many good books have already been written covering the benefits of exercise in those areas.

Just be aware that once you start exercising to sharpen your mind, you may have to put up with an increase in tolerance for stress or more physical energy and increased libido. Hey, I didn't say exercise would be without side-effects!

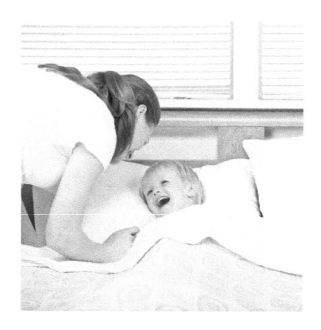

Chapter Fifty:
Sleep: Getting the Most Out of Bedtime

"Life is too short to sleep on low thread-count sheets."

- Leah Stussy.

Many people never really stop to think about the fact that close to 1/3 of their life will be spent in bed. When it comes to driving, the average person spends less than two hours a day in the car. That's less than ¼ the time they'll stretch out under the covers.

This fact alone was enough to get me to finally invest in the best mattress I could afford. After all, if we are going to borrow money for something that will depreciate the minute we drive it off the lot, wouldn't it make sense to have the same high standards on the square bag of stuffing we'll spend a good chunk of our life lying on?

Remember, we're no longer looking for the "Holy Grail"; I'm not proposing that your ADD/ADHD symptoms will suddenly disappear because you are sleeping on a mattress that allows you to adjust the air pressure to suit you. I am, however, suggesting that the research is conclusive regarding the connection between our health and the quality of the sleep we get - or don't.

From research, we've known for over twenty years, now, that sleep deprivation makes it very difficult to learn, and we also know that not getting enough sleep can cause challenges with focusing, make us tired (who would have guessed?) and put us on edge, causing us to have a "hair trigger" reaction to stressful events and to become irritable much more easily.

Here's something that might not be as obvious, to most. Studies from some of the nation's top sleep laboratories have concluded that many children who are tagged with the "ADD" label may simply be suffering from some level of sleep deprivation, and might find a near miraculous disappearance of their ADD symptoms from getting enough shut eye.

Shockingly, as much as 50% of the children diagnosed with ADHD experience sleep related problems. This is not limited to children, however, and sleep studies reveal that quality of sleep is a significant challenge for adults as well.

Below you will find some proven methods for getting the most out of your nocturnal hours ensuring that you are getting quality sleep.

Go to Bed and Get Up at the Same Time Each Day: It won't take long, and you'll find your body responding in a near Pavlovian manner. If you are going to make 11:00

pm your bedtime, then go to bed at 11:00 pm. If you are going to make 6:30 am your "Rise and Shine" time, then get up and going at 6:30 am. It's not rocket science, but the results you feel after just 2 - 3 weeks might convince you that it was.

Create a Pre-Sleep Ritual: Each time a fighter pilot climbs into a jet, no matter how long they've been flying, they always go through the exact pre-flight check that they did the time before. Why? One reason is the fact that each step of the checklist primes them for the task at hand, and the frame of mind that will be required. Likewise, by having a ritual or checklist of sorts that you go through each and every night, you'll be training your brain to guide itself into a good restful sleep.

Drown Out Distracting Noise: In short, "white noise" is any sound that helps you to sleep through sounds that would likely disturb your sleep otherwise.

Whether that white noise is generated by a simple box fan, or one of the many hi-tech machines on the market, the ability to keep those annoying noises from penetrating thd environment is sure to enhance your nighttime ventures.

Sniff Your Way to "La La Land": The sense of smell is perhaps the most powerful of the known five. Any smell that passes by your nostrils gets directly pumped into the brain, unlike the other senses that first pass through processing "stations".

Many scents and aromas have been shown to create a more "drowsy" feeling, helping prepare your brain for the transition into deep sleep. Lavender and chamomile are two that are sure to please.

"Zonin" with Melatonin: Have you ever noticed that you tend to get sleepy earlier in the winter months? If so, one likely reason is that your brain (pineal gland) produces more melatonin when the days are shorter. The length and intensity of daylight play a huge role in melatonin production.

By supplementing with melatonin, you can actually reset your body's internal clock, and ease into a restful sleep earlier in the evening, if you choose, or simply make your current bedtime more beneficial. In one study, those who were taking Ritalin were given melatonin. As a result, they fell asleep much more easily and quickly each evening.

Dim the Lights Early: You did read about melatonin, right? When you still have every lights in the house on at midnight, or are sitting in front of a glaring computer monitor when the ten o clock news comes on, as far as your brain is concerned, it's still day light. As a result, when you finally do shut the lights off (2 minutes before getting into bed) your pineal gland is playing a futile game of catch up.

Turn down the lights as early in the evening as you can, and you may just find that you are naturally getting sleepy much earlier, and sleeping much better when you do hit the sack.

Invest in Your Rest: Take a moment to add up how many hours you spend in your car each day. My guess is that it's far less than 6 - 8 hours. Most people will think nothing of financing a $40,000 vehicle, and yet, the very same people are often sleeping on an inferior mattress.

When you compare the time you spend in your car with the time you are in bed, it makes the 1 - 3 thousand dollars you will invest in a high quality mattress seem fairly insignificant.

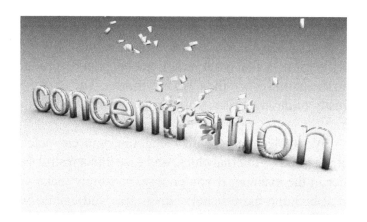

Chapter Fifty One:
The "How" of Creating New Habits
They Never Share with You

A man who gives his children habits of industry provides
for them better than by giving them fortune.

- Richard Whately

You've no doubt been told "It pays to develop good habits!" or something along those lines. The challenge with that, for most of us, is that as brilliant as this advice sounds, very few people ever tell us "how" to develop new and improved habits.

My hunch is that you've embarked on several plans to change an old habit, or create a new one before-with good intentions, but find that most of them didn't stick. As they say, "The road to hell is paved with good intentions!"

In this chapter, I'm going to hand you the "how"; the strategies that will make your transition from one way of behaving, to another, as easy and effective as it can be.

Link Things: I often have clients tell me "I know taking pycnogenol will probably help me, but I just never remember to take it!" This is a clear signal that they are trying to create a new habit, by taking the "add something new to my routine" approach.

Instead, why not link it to something that you already do every day? I'll bet you brush your teeth everyday (at least I'm hoping); why not place your pycnogenol next to your toothbrush or toothpaste? Doing this makes it seem more like an extension of something you've been doing for years, instead of something new. You can use this strategy for almost any habit you'd like to create. The question is "What do I already do, that I could link something to?"

See Yourself Doing It: Have you ever heard someone say "I just can't see myself doing that!"? As simplistic as it sounds, THAT may very well be the problem-literally. Think of anything that you already do every day.

Chances are very good, that you can easily see, or imagine yourself doing that in your mind. Now, think of something that you don't do everyday-yet. You'll likely find that it you can't yet imagine yourself doing that behavior as easily.

Whatever the new behavior is, take a couple of minutes, once or twice a day, to simply close your eyes and imagine yourself doing the behavior, at a certain place or time. (The place and time you desire this habit to manifest in your day to day life.)

Hardwire It: Many people have heard the "You establish a new habit in 21 days" advice. But let me ask you, don't you know several people-yourself included-that tried this approach, and still didn't get the habit to stick? There is a good reason for this; new research shows that to really "hardwire" new behaviors in, and make them resistant to change, we need to do them for 90 days.

Yes, after 21 days, you'll find you are more easily able to remember or do a new behavior, but it will still be vulnerable to reverting back to the old habit if you allow your focus to let up at this point. Keep a chart, checking off the new behavior each day, for 90 straight days. You'll like the result.

Make It Worthwhile: Incorporate the reward circuitry of your brain. When you do anything, and experience something pleasurable while you are doing it, or very soon thereafter, you radically increase the likeliness of this behavior occurring again.

How effective is this? Here's an example of what could be done with this strategy. If you and I were talking, face to face, and every time you took a sip of your coffee, I smiled at you, I could literally cause you to want to sip coffee when you were with me. A smile is processed as a sign of acceptance-a very good feeling to experience. In short, I would be linking the sipping of coffee, with the feeling acceptance.

What if every time you worked in a focused manner for 20 minutes, you allowed yourself to sniff a very pleasing aroma, like a comforting essential oil? What if every time you exercised, you allowed yourself to take a hot bath? (Meaning that on the days you skipped exercise, you could only shower)

By using your very creative mind, you can come up with countless ways you can reward yourself to make a new habit "take".

Now, you have the four critical "hows" of creating any new habit you desire. As you look back on the times you've tried, but failed, to create a new habit, you'll find that one or more of these crucial elements were missing.

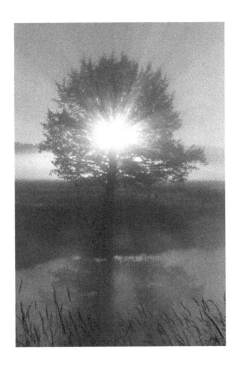

Chapter Fifty Two:
The Wisdom of Starting and Ending
Your Day with Peace

"Be pleasant until ten o'clock in the morning and the rest of the day will take care of itself."

- Elbert Hubbard.

In the field of psychology, the concepts of "Primacy" and "Recency" are well known. In short, we tend to remember, more than anything else, how something begins, and how it ends. Every professional speaker worth his or her weight in salt, knows that if nothing else, you'd better at least open and close your talk with a bang, and if you've ever been to a rock concert, you know they start the show, and do the encore with some of their best known songs.

Take just a moment and think about yesterday; I'll bet you can tell me about the first 30 - 60 minutes, and the last 30 - 60 minutes of your day with ease. For most people, though, the stuff in the middle starts to get a little fuzzy.

Since you already have this inherent ability to easily remember the first and last part of your day, you'd might as well use this inescapable fact to your advantage. See, most people leap out of bed at the last possible minute each morning, already behind the 8 ball, thinking about all of the things they have to do once they get to work, etc.

Then, at the end of the day, they replay the day's most stressful events in their mind getting as many stress hormones flowing as they can, just before they drift off for a not so restful sleep.

Why not begin and end your day with calm, peace and relaxation? I often use the sandwich metaphor to describe the impact of this. If you have a nice lean beef hamburger... with two hard and stale pieces of bread or bun, it's really hard to enjoy what's in the middle. If you start and end your day in a stressful way, it's really hard to enjoy much of what happens in between.

One of the best ways I know of for starting your day with peace is to get up 1 hour earlier than you have to. I know, I know... you may be thinking *"ugggghhhh... I can barely get up the way it is now!"* Just remember, once you begin employing some of the other ideas in this book, your energy level is going to lift.

By getting up an hour early, you get to enjoy the feeling of doing nothing, of sipping tea or coffee, or watching the sun come up. There is a calm that must be experienced to be appreciated that happens with this ritual; a calm that will carry over into the rest of the day.

In the evening, carve out 30 - 60 minutes where you shut off all sources of external information, and allow your mind to roam, to think any thoughts that flit through your mind, and if you are going to reflect on the day, reflect on all of the things you are grateful for that you have experienced.

If you'll stick with the morning/evening ritual for a week, you'll do it for a month, and if you do it for a month, I'm betting that you'll do it for the rest of your life... it's that profound.

About the Author

Dr. Clare Albright is a Clinical Psychologist in Lake Forest, CA.

She has been counseling in Orange County, CA for 30 years, and is the proud mother of a 14 year old son.

Dr. Albright has been a public speaker for over three decades and is available to speak with your group about:

- Attention Deficit Disorder and ADHD
- Parenting
- Staying Close to Your Child
- Positive Child Discipline
- Parenting Adolescents
- Anxiety Disorders
- Neurofeedback Therapy
- Biofeedback Therapy
- Stress Management

Dr. Albright will 'wow' your group with her warm, humorous, educational and inspiring presentation.

Dr. Albright is a graduate of Coach University and provides life coaching services by telephone and Skype all over the globe.

Dr. Albright can be reached at (949) 454-0996.